TRADITIONAL
Thai Medicine

TRADITIONAL Thai Medicine

Buddhism, Animism, Ayurveda

C. PIERCE SALGUERO

HOHM PRESS

Cover design: Kim Johansen
Layout and design: Zachary Parker, Kadak Graphics

Library of Congress Cataloging in Publication Data:

Salguero, C. Pierce.
 Traditional Thai medicine : Buddhism, animism, ayurveda / C. Pierce Salguero.
 p. ; cm.
 Includes bibliographical references.
 ISBN-13: 978-1-890772-67-3 (pbk. : alk. paper)
 ISBN-10: 1-890772-67-4 (pbk. : alk. paper)
 1. Traditional medicine--Thailand--History. I. Title.
 [DNLM: 1. Medicine, Oriental Traditional--Thailand. WB 50 JT3 S164t 2007]
 R611.T45S26 2007
 615.8'809593--dc22
 2006101568

HOHM PRESS
P.O. Box 2501
Prescott, AZ 86302
800-381-2700
http://www.hohmpress.com

This book was printed in the U.S.A. on recycled, acid-free paper using soy ink.

5   4   3   2   1

Acknowledgements

This book is dedicated to the generations of teachers who have contributed to the practice of traditional Thai medicine. Specifically, I want to thank my own teachers, the late Ajahn Sintorn Chaichakan, Ajahn Wasan, Ajahn Pramost, "Mama" Lek Chaiya Thiwong, Pikul Termyod, and all of the others who pointed the way for me in the long gestation of this project. I also want to thank the many named and anonymous readers of this manuscript who helped with its evolution—especially Wit Sukhsamran, whose insights and valuable suggestions have made this a much better book, and whose generosity and friendship have been most welcome. Last but not least, I wish to thank my own students of Thai healing arts who have taken up this knowledge with enthusiasm, and who continue its practice with respect and integrity.

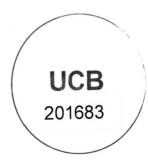

Contents

Timeline for History of Medicine in Thailand

India

4th–3rd century B.C.E.	Lifetime of Siddhatta Gotama (the Buddha) and Jivaka Komarabhacca
273-237 B.C.E.	King Ashoka
1st century B.C.E.	Earliest Buddhist texts written
100 B.C.E.-500 C.E.	Mahayana Buddhism emerges
by 300 C.E.	*Caraka Samhita* reaches current form
by 500 C.E.	*Sushruta Samhita* reaches current form
700-1100 C.E.	Buddhist and Hindu Tantra flourishes

Thailand

400-600 C.E.	Theravada Buddhism arrives
800 C.E.	T'ai migrations from Tonkin underway
1238	Sukothai established
1351	Ayutthaya established
1657-1688	Reign of King Narai
1687-88	de la Loubère in Siam
1765-1767	Burmese sack Ayutthaya
1782	King Rama I crowned and est. Bangkok
1789-1801	Wat Pho rebuilt as royal temple
1830s	Medical tablets and statues created
1908	First publication of herbal texts
1957	Wat Pho medical school established
1973	Shivagakomarpaj Hospital established by Ajahn Sintorn Chaichakan
1978	WHO directive encourages government support of local medical traditions

Introduction

Traditional Thai medicine[1] is an officially recognized healing system alongside modern Western biomedicine and Traditional Chinese Medicine in Thailand today. Traditional doctors (*mo boran* or *mo phaen boran*), as defined by the government, are those "practicing the healing arts by means of knowledge gained from traditional texts or study which is not based on science." This definition stands in contradistinction to biomedical doctors, whose training *is* based on science.[2]

The paths to medical licensure in each of these arenas are comparable, but quite separate. Every formally-trained TTM practitioner is required by the government to study a standardized curriculum, which typically includes one year of classes to become a traditional pharmacist and another two years to become a full physician. The arts of therapeutic massage (*nuad boran* or *nuad phaen boran*) or traditional midwifery (*pradung kahn*) can be taken during a fourth, optional, year. Students graduating from these programs are examined by the Ministry of Public Health, and are licensed and regulated by the national government through a process parallel to that which regulates medical doctors, nurses, and other practitioners of Western medicine.

A study in 2005 counted 37,157 practitioners in various branches of TTM,[3] and reported that 83.3 percent of hospitals,

---

1 The government of Thailand and some academic work use the abbreviation TTM.
2 Mulholland (1979c), p. 224.
3 This total represented 14,912 practitioners in "Thai traditional medicine," 18,997 in "Thai traditional pharmacy," 2,869 in "Thai traditional midwifery," and 379 "applied Thai traditional medicine practitioners." See Chokevivat (2005), p. 4.

67.8 percent of community centers, and 22.4 percent of health centers incorporated TTM to some degree.[4] Despite a high level of official support and popularity in modern times, however, traditional medicine in Thailand has never received much Western academic attention. There was some initial interest among certain Europeans—mostly missionaries—in the nineteenth and early twentieth centuries. Unfortunately, much of what was written during this period was condescending and racist, resulting from a colonial mentality and a bent toward "civilizing the savages" with Western medicine and Protestant Christianity.[5]

Western scholarly interest took off only after the rediscovery of Southeast Asia as a result of the Vietnam War. Many academics wrote books and dissertations in the 1970s and 1980s on Thailand, including several on Thai medicine. Important scholars from this period include Somchintana Ratarasarn and Jean Mulholland, who analyzed the authoritative texts taught at the licensed medical schools, Louis Golomb and Ruth Inge-Heinze, who tackled the shadowy world of Thai exorcists and magical healers, and Viggo Brun and Trond Schumacher, who undertook the study of rural herbalism. These scholars contributed enormously to our knowledge about Thai medicine, but their passion unfortunately did not extend to the next generation of academics and the field of Thai traditional medical studies appears to have been a non-starter. There are currently very few Western scholars writing on this subject.

Traditional Thai medicine is diverse and complicated. In reviewing the existing literature, one receives the impression that there are in fact two separate Thai medical systems—the scholarly practices based on Ayurveda and centered around the *mo boran*, and a very different tradition based among poor illiterate rural healers. Several scholars, particularly Brun and Schumacher,[6] have characterized this split as a dichotomy between "royal"

4 Chokevivat (2005), p. 6.
5 See Bradley (1967) for a good example of this type of literature.
6 Brun and Schumacher (1994).

medicine, or a literate form of medicine practiced at the court among learned doctors, and "rural" medicine, or the eclectic practices of the village. However, other scholars, such as Hinderling and Golomb, have demonstrated that so-called "rural" practices are just as popular in the modern cities, and therefore reject the notion of an urban-rural bifurcation.[7] Heinze's work has instead referred to a split between "elite" and "folk" medicine,[8] but this convention still promotes the view that there are two separate traditions of healing.

More recent scholarship in the history of European and East Asian culture has emphasized that applying such labels imposes a bias on academic research. However, for organizational purpose I will utilize these terms here in a limited way. My approach in this book will be to look into the historical context for medicine in Thailand in Part I; the literate "elite" tradition of TTM in Part II; and "folk" or non-literate medicine in Part III. I hope in this way to present a balanced approach to both the history and the modern practice of Thai medicine while acknowledging both its roots and its diversity.

Parts II and III do approach seemingly different bodies of medical knowledge. "Elite" Thai medicine includes practices heavily influenced by India, which I refer to in this book as Thai Ayurveda (for herbal practices) and Thai Yoga (for physical regimen). Although there are some differences, much of the theory of textually-based Thai herbal prescription is in fact based on the Indian Ayurvedic *Caraka* and *Sushruta Samhitas*. As I will show, the written material from the Bangkok period is largely derived of Ayurvedic origin. Traditional Thai massage and physical exercises likewise are closely related to Indian *hatha-yoga*. These practices together form the basis of the system that is taught at the authoritative schools and that is regulated by the government today. Thus "elite" Thai medicine self-consciously looks to the

---

7   Hinderling (1973) and Golomb (1985).
8   Heinze (1992).

Indian medical classics as its foundational literature and incorporates much of this theoretical background.

However, any analysis of Thai medicine must not only focus on the Ayurvedic and yogic influences, but must also discuss the ways in which non-Indian ideas are implemented in daily practice by Thai healers. In fact, "folk" practices based on indigenous T'ai animism,[9] popular Buddhist ritual, Chinese medicine, and Tantric cabalism are found throughout Thailand and remain extremely popular today, despite the fact that they are largely ignored in the medical literature and are therefore typically relegated to the realm of "folk" medicine. These diverse practices are mentioned throughout the text, but will be discussed in detail in Part III.

Though I apportion the book in this way, it will become clear that I am of the opinion that there are very few traditional healers (or patients) who can be pigeon-holed into one or another category. While recognizing that in some cases it may be useful to distinguish between an elite and a non-literate tradition, I have come to believe from my own research and field study that healing in Thailand is better approached as a diverse collection of very different practices that resist easy classification. As a model for understanding and speaking about Thai medicine, I prefer to keep the categorization of practices and ideas messy rather than use the unity implied by the government label "TTM" or the duality implied by the "elite-folk" split. I believe that a single label over-simplifies the diversity of Thai medicine and misleadingly implies there is a single theoretical system. But, the impression that there are two Thai medicines may be equally misleading in that it implies a strict dichotomy.

In practice, however, the Thai government, and practitioners themselves, utilize this "two-medicines" model when elite physicians or official ministries differentiate between licensed and

---

9   Note that in this book I use the conventions "T'ai" to refer to the ancient ethnic group that is scattered throughout Southeast Asia, "Siamese" to refer to the T'ai kingdoms of Siam, and "Thai" to refer to the residents of the modern nation Thailand.

unlicensed healers. This divide is reinforced and maintained by scholarship when researchers from different disciplines look at Thai tradition through differently-colored academic lenses. The analysis of Thai "folk" medicine has usually been undertaken by anthropologists, who spend long periods of time in field study with practitioners, usually in remote villages. On the other hand, the analysis of written texts and other artifacts has usually been the purview of the historian. Thai medical texts tend to belong squarely to the "elite" tradition, and for the most part prioritize Thailand's Indian heritage over the various other practices.

I have attempted in this book to bridge these two approaches by incorporating the work of both historians and anthropologists. I believe that medicine in Thailand is best approached as a "medical marketplace" in which practitioners of many different stripes offer diverse products and services based on different models of disease and the body. "Elite" Thai medicine as taught at the government-recognized traditional medical schools is one ingredient in the marketplace. The village shamaness using eggs to exorcise ghosts from her patients is another. The Buddhist monk offering protection rituals, the magical tattoo artist, and the bone-setter each contributes to this marketplace as well.

This book will show that there are different views of body and self co-existing simultaneously in Thailand today. These views arise from the influences of Theravada Buddhism, Ayurveda, yoga, Chinese medicine, indigenous T'ai beliefs, and other influences, and are brought together in unique and idiosyncratic ways by individual practitioners. Although there are some central ideas that permeate throughout the medical community, no two practitioners are alike in every way. At this point in the scholarship of Thai medicine, it is unclear what determines individual patients' decisions in the marketplace. What types of healers are sought out undoubtedly is influenced by a complex and idiosyncratic blend of economic, social, cultural, political, and institutional factors that anthropologists and sociologists have yet to adequately explore.

The few studies of this nature are hopelessly outdated, and this topic awaits serious investigation.[10]

The situation among Thai patients may be understood by the following metaphor, used by the medical anthropologist, Arthur Kleinman, to describe popular culture in Taiwan.[11] We can imagine that the medical field in Thailand is a dim-sum restaurant, in which waiters circulate carrying trays of food. While the food is circulating around the room, patients help themselves to what they like from the trays. Although the food is all coming out of the same kitchen, each customer winds up with a unique meal. Analogously, although there are some consistencies throughout the medical field, the practices and influences each patient selects from the offered options is likely to be different. The range of practices offered by different healers the patient comes in contact with can be similarly unique. The result is that medicine is highly unique and personal, both for those providing and those consuming healthcare. While this presents certain challenges for the scholar of Thai medicine, this diversity is in fact an acknowledged and desirable feature of traditional Thai medicine, valued by those who patronize this system in their daily lives.[12]

In this study, I will look at sources that reflect many of these various viewpoints. Chief among the ancient sources will be the Pali canon, the foundational texts of the Theravada Buddhist tradition (committed to writing in Sri Lanka in the first century B.C.E., but for the most part composed in previous centuries in India and transmitted orally). I will also refer to several Ayurvedic compendia, most importantly the *Caraka* and *Sushruta Samhitas* (compiled in current form c. 300 C.E. and 500 C.E. respectively), which are commonly considered to be among the most important texts in the Indian tradition, and which are part of the foundation of Thai medicine as well. I will also bring in

10 I cite Golomb (1985) and Hinderling (1973) in this book as the most recent studies. I am unaware of any updates to their work.
11 Kleinman (1980), p. 96.
12 Golomb (1985), p. 146.

indigenous Thai texts, most notably the *Thai Book of Genesis* (date unknown), which has been translated by Mulholland and is the only complete canonical medical text I know of available in English.[13] (A complete table of contents of the Thai medical canon is presented in Appendix A.)

The main modern written source for this book is the student manual in use in 1997 by the Shivagakomarpaj Traditional Medicine Hospital. This is a traditional clinic and medical school in northern Thailand which is in many ways at the center of the "elite-folk" debate, as it is both a government-licensed medical school and a community clinic offering free traditional healthcare to the surrounding villages, self-consciously incorporating local medical knowledge into the national curriculum. In the current book, I will use translations of Shivagakomarpaj's basic herbal manual I made with the assistance of two practitioners while conducting field research, and will also draw upon its manual of massage therapy, supplemented by information from my notes taken while attending Shivagakomarpaj's classes.

In order to give a more balanced overview of Thai medicine, and to incorporate the non-literate practices, I will contextualize these written sources by looking at various so-called folk practices and their implementation in the modern day. For the most part, I will rely on my own ethnographic observations made during the periods I apprenticed in traditional Thai healing while living in Chiang Mai for twenty-six months between 1997 and 2001, supplemented by secondary sources from the field of anthropology.

My own training in Thai medicine was undertaken in phases with many different known and not so well-known teachers over a relatively wide span of time. However, my main *ajahns* (masters) were Lek Chaiya Thiwong, a charismatic individual with whom I spent much time on the living room floor learning herbal practices, and the late Sintorn Chaichakan, the founder of the

13 Mulholland (1989).

Shivagakomarpaj Traditional Medicine Hospital, at which I sojourned as a student and, later, as a substitute teacher.

Despite bringing these new sources and observations into the conversation, I am not looking to break much new academic ground in this current project. My intent in this book is only to summarize the existing English-language scholarship on Thai medicine, and to point the way for future research (which, I might add, is sorely needed). I should warn readers that this book is not intended as a comprehensive overview of the history or anthropology of Thailand. I would suggest that those interested in more detailed analysis refer to the overviews provided by Tarling (1992) and Lockard (1995) for history and Bowen (1995) for anthropology, but as is the case with any dynamic academic discipline, I know that almost as soon as I write these words, these suggestions will become obsolete—if they have not already done so. Another note to the reader: as I do not read Thai, I will not be including the scholarship in that language. I also will not pay attention to standardization of Thai transcription practices, and will in many cases spell words as they are spelled in the literature I am quoting and citing.

It is clear that this book is just a beginning. It is my sincere hope that, despite its shortcomings, it may inspire practitioners of Thai healing arts as well as future scholars to look at Thai medicine more seriously as a field of study. In my presentation of this material, I also hope I may have made some small contribution to the tradition my Thai teachers have graciously shared with me. As is traditional to say on these occasions: any credit due is due to them for their selfless interest in my training and willingness to share their wisdom; any shortcomings in my presentation or understanding are mine alone.

PART I

The Historical Context

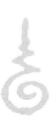

CHAPTER 1

A Historical Review of Medicine in Pre-Modern Siam

Early T'ai Migrations[1]

According to research in linguistics, genetics, and anthropology, the T'ais are believed to have inhabited a homeland in the Tonkin region on the coast of modern Vietnam. Due to population pressures, they are believed to have begun migrating into the modern Chinese province of Yunnan at some unknown point no later than the eighth century C.E.[2] It was not until the twelfth century that the T'ais moved south as well, into modern Laos, Thailand, Burma, and Assam. Pockets of T'ai people continue to inhabit this large geographic area today, where they are known locally as Tai (in Vietnam), Dai (in Southern China), or Thai (in Thailand).

Indianization of Southeast Asia had begun in earnest in the first centuries of the Common Era.[3] By the twelfth century, Indic culture had spread from modern Cambodia to the islands of Indonesia. Before the arrival of the T'ais, the region that would be called Siam (also Syam or Sayam) was dominated by the

---

1 This chapter does not intend to provide a comprehensive history of pre-modern Thailand. The reader should refer to Tarling (1992) for this purpose.
2 See Terwiel (1978a) for a discussion of origins and early T'ai migrations.
3 Tarling (1992), p. 281.

Mon kingdom of Dvaravati (fl. sixth to twelfth centuries) and the Khmer Empire (fl. seventh to eleventh centuries). Indian and Chinese merchants plied this area continually. Political boundaries throughout the region were fluid, power frequently changed hands, and a diversity of people competed for the region's rich economic resources. Thus, the T'ais moved into a region characterized by cultural and political diversity.

Once they settled in modern day Thailand, the influences on T'ai culture continued to be varied. Theravada Buddhism probably entered from the northwestern Dvaravati (in modern-day Burma).[4] Theravada, or "the Teachings of the Elders," is a form of Buddhism based on a conservative interpretation of the earliest Buddhist texts. From the little surviving evidence of the Dvaravati kingdom (limited largely to archaeological evidence such as coins and sculpture[5]), historians believe that it had close connections with other Theravada kingdoms in South Asia, particularly the Sinhalese kingdoms in modern Sri Lanka. The Siamese T'ais are thought to have converted to Theravada Buddhism under Dvaravati influence shortly after their arrival in the area.[6]

But this was not the only influence on the T'ai people. Mahayana Buddhism and Brahmanism were also formidable Indian influences across Southeast Asia.[7] Despite the dominance of Theravada Buddhism, aspects of these other traditions have to this day been retained in Thai art, architecture, and folk belief. To this day, most Thai temples include in their iconography Indian deities such as Hanuman, Ganesha and Garuda (although these are invariably placed in positions subservient to the Theravada icons). The *Ramakien*, the national epic of Thailand, is none other than the familiar Indian story of the *Ramayana*, which has provided centuries of South and Southeast Asian artisans and storytellers with a source of inspiration (not to mention also inspiring the names of both the

---

4   Tarling (1992), p. 295.
5   See examples of Dvaravati art from Thailand in Fischer (1993).
6   Griswold and Nagara (1975), p. 32.
7   See Tarling (1992), pp. 286-304.

kingdom of Ayutthaya and the reign-titles of the modern line of Kings named "Rama"). Unlike in the Hindu tradition, where these figures are all-powerful deities, in Thailand, due to the primacy of Theravada, they are *thewada*, or demigods subservient to and "pacified" by the Buddha. Although they can become wrathful if angered, these gods are frequently "channeled" by spirit mediums who have special relationships with the unseen world, and can be called upon for information or protection in time of need.

The Sukothai Kingdom

In 1238, the T'ai ruler Si Intharathit established Sukothai ("Dawn of Happiness") in what is now northern Thailand, and began to exercise control over this previously Khmer territory.[8] The Sukothai period is considered by Thais to be the "Golden Age" of Siam, and the third king, Ramakhamhaeng (or "Rama the Brave") is said to have been among the most benevolent and righteous in Siamese history.[9]

At Sukothai, the T'ais seem to have begun what would be a long tradition of eclecticism, incorporating social, political, and cultural ideas from these many sources. However, according to historians A.B. Griswold and Prasert Na Nagara, when compared with later Siamese kingdoms, Sukothai was also perhaps the most T'ai.[10] During this period, according to Griswold and Nagara, the fundamental principles of ethics were established which would influence Siamese law and government over the succeeding centuries, and the T'ais began to experiment with the institutions of statecraft. The basis for the modern Thai script was developed as well at this time.

Inscriptions from Sukothai are regrettably few, the tropical climate and centuries of war having exacted their toll on the

8   Tarling (1992), p. 169.
9   Griswold and Nagara (1975), pp. 43-44. Recent scholarship considers much of Ramakhamhaeng's legacy to be legendary.
10 Griswold and Nagara (1975), p. 67.

material record. Nevertheless, although none remain from this period, it could have been at this time that the first Siamese medical treatises were recorded. The evidence we do have of medical activity in this period is limited to a stone inscription from a neighboring Khmer king, Chaivoraman, that mentions the existence of 102 hospitals called *arogaya sala* established throughout the kingdom, including in the Khmer-held region that today is northeastern Thailand.[11]

Medical Texts from the Ayutthaya Period

Ayutthaya, a T'ai kingdom founded in 1351 in what is today central Thailand, annexed Sukothai in 1376. Extending into the Khmer regions of Lopburi and U Thong, Ayutthaya became the dominant T'ai kingdom in the region until its fall in the eighteenth century (other important T'ai kingdoms included Lan Na around modern-day Chiang Mai, and the Lao cities along the middle Mekong River).[12]

Although Ayutthaya was founded by a T'ai ruler named Ramathibodhi I, most of its territory had long been under Khmer influence, and the new state was more heavily influenced by the Brahmanic government rituals and Hinduized religion of the Khmers than Sukothai had been.[13] Perhaps because it was established as a center for trade rather than agriculture, Ayutthaya became one of the most successful and cosmopolitan cities in the region.[14]

By all accounts, Ayutthaya was a vibrant and wealthy place. Many ethnic groups coexisted in the busy ports and markets of the Ayutthaya kingdom. The ideas that developed in this milieu were, not surprisingly, eclectic and syncretic. Though scant, what historical evidence remains tell us that, reflecting their society

11 Chokevivat and Chuthaputti (2005), p. 4.
12 Tarling (1992), p. 171.
13 Griswold and Nagara (1975), p. 67.
14 Hodges (1998), p. 82.

more generally, Ayutthayan medicine was also multicultural.

The Ayutthayan medical system was probably not borrowed in its entirety from a previously existing tradition, nor was it necessarily adopted all at once. Indian forms of medicine probably entered Sukothai and Ayutthaya along with other Indic cultural influences from a diversity of sources. As we will see, material from Theravada, Ayurveda, and yoga all would influence medical tradition. However, the knowledge the T'ais brought with them also remained a major factor, and even today indigenous beliefs continue to form an important layer of cosmology and healing among modern T'ai people across Southeast Asia.[15] Contact with Muslim communities, Chinese merchants, Hindu traders, and even European explorers and missionaries during the Ayutthaya period also can not be ignored.

Ayutthaya was ultimately destroyed when the city was burned and looted by Burmese invaders from 1765 to 1767. The devastation left the economy in shambles, toppled the reigning dynasty, and threatened to end the state altogether. Due to the near-complete destruction, we are left with very few texts or other primary materials relating to Ayutthayan medicine. However, at least one important medical text is extant. This text, the *Tamraa phra osot Phra Narai* (*Medical Texts of King Narai*), is a small book which collects a number of herbal prescriptions said to have been presented to King Narai (1657-1688) and to his successor King Phettharatcha (1688-1697).

King Narai himself is an interesting figure. In the Ayutthaya King Narai's time, the temple was the seat of education for art, law, history, philosophy, astrology, mathematics, and medicine.[16] The sciences were taught by Brahmins in a traditional model, but King Narai was unusually interested in Western knowledge. During his reign he sought out, and received as gifts from European dignitaries, scientific instruments. However, because

---

15 See Terwiel (1978a).
16 Information in this section from Hodges (1998), p. 87-90.

this interest was restricted to himself, the impact of Western ideas on Siamese society seems to have been quite limited. It would not be until the reign of Rama IV in the Bangkok period that Western science, and medicine in particular, would make a larger impact on Thai society.

The herbal manuscript does not betray a sign of this Western influence, but rather seems to belong to an older indigenous tradition of herbal prescription. Mulholland briefly describes this text in her outline of the history of Thai medical documents.[17] Mulholland writes that the names and dates cited within the document, and the bamboo manuscript itself, indicate that these recipes were in use in the latter seventeenth and early eighteenth centuries. Inscribed on palm-leaf manuscripts in the eighteenth century, these prescriptions were subsequently found by the medical expert and professor, Prince Damrong Rajanubhap, in the Royal Library and were compiled for publication for the first time in 1917 as part of a cremation text commemorating the death of a well-known Bangkok physician. The *Medical Texts of King Narai* was apparently a highly valued collection. Many similar texts were owned by the royal family and the royal physicians, but the name and the contents of this particular manuscript imply that this was King Narai's personal collection of prescriptions. This manuscript was also apparently used as a textbook of recipes.[18]

The palm leaf manuscripts of King Narai are representative of a fundamental feature of Thai medicine remarked upon by Brun and Schumacher: the importance of special herbal recipes handed down through generations of healers.[19] This type of manuscript typically comprises a list of individual recipes written on palm leaves and bound together within bamboo covers. According to Brun and Schumacher, these fragile texts are highly valued, and can represent the traditional doctor's most potent healing tool.

17 Mulholland (1987), p. 7-19.
18 Chokevivat and Chuthaputti (2005), p. 4.
19 Brun and Schumacher (1994), p. 44.

The texts are often passed from teacher to student as a set, though each prescription is used separately in practice. These individual prescriptions are often traded among practitioners, who continually seek to acquire more, sometimes by traveling quite widely. The efficacy of a given healer may be measured by the number of prescriptions he possesses, although modern herbalists typically use a handful of especially revered recipes for treatment of most diseases.

Among those who utilize them today, Brun and Schumacher report that these texts are accorded veneration equal to Buddhist *suttas*, or other sacred texts. This is consistent with findings from earlier periods. Daniel Beach Bradley, an American missionary doctor writing in 1865, noted of the medical manuscripts common to his day, "there is a similar air of sanctity thrown over Siamese medical books, as there is over their religious books; and almost as soon would they discredit the latter as the former."[20] Today, these types of manuscripts are typically found among folk herbalists, and no longer play much of a role in the formal TTM system, which relies heavily on printed materials and published books for the preservation and transmission of medical knowledge.[21]

There are no other complete medical texts definitively datable to the Ayutthaya era discussed in the English academic literature other than the King Narai manuscript. However, an important early primary source that is well-known is an eyewitness account of Siamese culture and customs written by Simon de la Loubère, a French envoy who visited for four months from 1687-88. His work was published in France in 1691 under the title *Du Royaume de Siam*, and republished in English in 1693 as *The Kingdom of Siam*. Although he devotes little space to the practice of medicine—and what he writes is somewhat disparaging—de la Loubère includes several intriguing passages.

---

20 Bradley (1967), p. 83.
21 Brun and Schumacher (1994) discuss these manuscripts in the context of Northern Thai folk herbal traditions.

These passages hint at the character of Ayutthayan medicine. Firstly, de la Loubère mentions the existence of cherished herbal manuscripts such as those just described, and possibly refers to the passing of herbal recipes from teacher to student:

> [The Siamese] trouble not themselves to have any principle of Medicine, but only a number of Receipts, which they have learnt from their Ancestors, and in which they never alter a thing.[22]

More importantly, perhaps, is de la Loubère's description of the eclectic and multi-ethnic approach to medicine at the Siamese court:

> The King of Siam's principal Physicians are Chineses [sic]; and he has also some Siameses [sic] and Peguins [Mon]: and within two or three years he has admitted into this quality Mr. Panmart, of the French Secular Missionaries, on whom he relies more than on all his other Physicians. The others are obliged to report daily unto him the state of this Prince's health, and to receive from his hand the Remedies which he prepares for him.[23]

From this passage, one can infer that, as he wrote, de la Loubère was witnessing a moment in history when Siamese physicians were being replaced by foreign specialists. From these accounts, we can surmise that the Siamese court at Ayutthaya allowed a tolerant approach to medicine—pragmatism and syncretism being a recurring feature of T'ai culture in any era—not only allowing for the practice of medicine by foreigners, but employing foreign doctors in the service of the king. However, we should note that Indian physicians are conspicuously missing from de la Loubère's

---

22 de la Loubère (1969), p. 62.
23 de la Loubère (1969), p. 62.

list of practitioners. There is thus no indication in de la Loubère's writings that the court medicine of his time was dependent on Indian practitioners, although it is likely that the Siamese and Mon practitioners mentioned were knowledgeable of Ayurveda.

Medicine in the Bangkok Era

Our window onto early Siamese medicine is admittedly sketchy and vague. It is not until the Bangkok period that a detailed material record of traditional Thai medicine is found. However, from this point the materials are abundant. As outlined above, we really do not know much about Ayutthayan medicine, but what evidence is available (at least in the English-language sources) points toward a picture of an eclectic practice. But, as we will see, if Indian medicine was not hegemonic during the time that Loubère was at court, it certainly became a powerful national symbol in the nineteenth century and came to dominate modern TTM.

After the fall of Ayutthaya, a tumultuous power struggle saw the rise and fall of the notorious usurper Phraya Taksin (r. 1769-1782), who successfully recaptured territory in the North from the Burmese, and attempted to unite the kingdom behind his capital at Thonburi, across the river from modern-day Bangkok.[24] Taksin, who history records as a cruel ruler who imagined himself to be the Buddha incarnate, was eventually dethroned and executed. His general, Chao Phrya Chakri, assumed the Thai kingship in 1782. Posthumously named King Rama I (r. 1782-1809), the founder of the Chakri dynasty was legendary already in his own lifetime for having captured the Emerald Buddha, the most valued Buddhist icon in Siam, from the Lao in 1779.

Within fifteen days of his coronation, Rama I established a capital across the river at Bangkok. There, he began a program of cultural revival with the intention to restore Siam to its former

---

24 Historical information in this section is from Terwiel (1983).

glory. The project began by constructing the new royal palace, which was not only a replica of Ayutthaya, but which utilized the actual bricks salvaged from the ruins of the old Siamese capital. This was an intentional symbolic act conveying not only Rama I's intention to rule as an Ayutthayan king, but also to affirm that the glorious Siam of days gone by was once again on the ascendant.

Much of Rama I's Siamese renaissance took place at the Wat Phra Chetuphon Wimon Mangkhalaram temple in Bangkok.[25] This temple, commonly known as Wat Pho, is known to have existed as a simple provincial monastery some time before 1688, and was originally named Wat Potharam (hence the modern nickname). When he moved the capital, Rama I established Wat Pho as the primary royal temple, and set out to rebuild and enlarge the facility. Construction at Wat Pho began in 1789 and was ultimately completed in April, 1801. The new royal temple was adjacent to the site of the king's Bangkok residence, and it was similarly constructed on the Ayutthayan model, and with equal grandeur.

Rama I also initiated an era of traditional medical revival.[26] He began to collect at Wat Pho traditional medical formulas and established the Department of Pharmacy (Khrom Mo Rong Phra Osoth) on the Ayutthayan model. His successor, Rama II, continued the efforts to gather medical texts from around the kingdom. In 1816, he passed the Royal Pharmacists Law, which enabled royal pharmacists to freely travel the kingdom in search of medicinal substances.

Wat Pho, the Medical Library in Stone

Only thirty-one years after the establishment of Wat Pho, the third Chakri king, Rama III (r. 1824-1851) began renovations and enlarged the temple's facilities yet again. At that time, he designated Wat Pho a "democratic university of comprehensive

25 See Matics (1979) for information on Wat Pho in these paragraphs.
26 Information in this paragraph from Wibulbolprasert (2005), Chapter 1.

education" designed to house a huge collection of artifacts from across the kingdom at that location.[27] In the words of his grandchild, Prince Dhani Nivat, King Rama III intended for Wat Pho to be the "seat of learning for all classes of people in all walks of life" which would "expound all branches of traditional knowledge, both religious and secular."[28] At a time when skills were traditionally handed down through the family, the king's effort to bring together the arts and sciences at this one educational facility was unprecedented.[29] As part of this project, the king ordered the compilation of the seminal texts of all the scholarly traditions of Siam and the development of authoritative textbooks in these various fields. Beginning in 1832, texts were etched into marble tablets and various sculptures were commissioned to permanently store this knowledge in a "library in stone."[30]

As one of the traditional sciences, medical materials were established on the grounds of Wat Pho at this time as well. These included statuaries with figures of *ruesri* (hermit-sages) constructed in 1836 by a kinsman of the king, Prince Nagara (*see Fig. 1*). Unfortunately, the original plan to execute the statues in metal did not come to pass, and the more perishable stucco was used. Thus, of the eighty statues first commissioned, only about a quarter of them have survived to today. Among these, there remains only a single example demonstrating massage.[31] The remaining depict individual yogic practice for therapeutic aims, a tradition known today as *ruesri dat ton* (or "hermit's self-stretching"). These statues are paired with inscriptions bearing instructions written by physicians, members of the royal family, government officials, monks, and even the king himself.[32]

---

27 Matics (1979), p. 43.
28 Nivat (1933), p. 143.
29 Matics (1979), p. 43.
30 Griswold (1965), p. 319.
31 Griswold (1965), p. 320.
32 Matics (1978), p. 254. These inscriptions eventually became separated from the images, but Griswold and Matics have both laboriously reunited the statues with their textual counterparts (see Griswold [1965] and Matics [1978]).

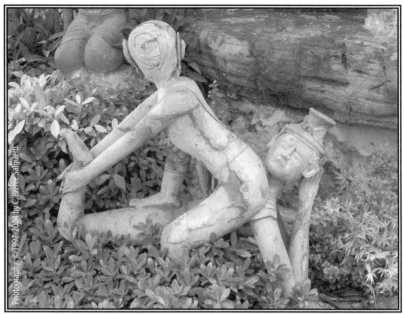

Photography ©1997–2004 by C. Pierre Salguero.

FIG. 1. THE ONLY REMAINING STATUES OF RUESRI PERFORMING TRADITIONAL MEDICAL MASSAGE. WAT PHO, BANGKOK.

A manuscript from 1838 which catalogued and explained the statues includes descriptive passages such as these:

> We are about to begin describing the system of posture exercises invented by experts to cure ailments and make them vanish away... Stretching out the arms and manipulating the fingers, while sitting with thighs raised upward, will relieve stiff arms. This Rishi (named) Yaga, adopts the cure called "The Four Ascetics Blended Together." The ascetic sitting on a crag with feet pointing downward is named Vyadhipralaya, of world-wide renown. He raises one hand, while massaging and squeezing his elbow with the other, a posture to dispel the stubborn indisposition that makes his feet and hand stiff, and to relax them.[33]

---

33 Griswold (1965), p. 321. See this article for more images and captions.

The manuscript continues likewise to describe other various postures and their therapeutic applications.

On the construction of these statues, the manuscript continues:

> [In 1836] the King gave the command to his kinsman Prince Goemamün... to assemble craftsmen... to cast statues of the Eighty Experts displaying the posture exercises. When the statues were finished and painted in color, they were set up in the proper sequence around [Wat Pho], accompanied by inscriptions on the walls giving the name of each one of them and their technique of curing ailments. All of this was done so as to be useful to people of every rank like a donation of medicine. Thus has His Majesty increased the store of His merits, and made His fame to shine until heaven and earth come to an end.[34]

These statues are examples of the importance of Indian medical knowledge in Bangkok-era Siam. The connections with Indian medicine are overt. These figures are portrayed wearing dhotis of the Indian style, with matted hair in the fashion of Hindu ascetics. Indian influence can also be seen in the appearance among these figures of Hanuman, a character from the popular adaptation of the Indian folk tale, the Ramayana (Th. Ramakien).[35]

The medical artifacts preserved at this "library in stone" also included numerous diagrams depicting pressure points and *sen* lines (more or less analogous to Indian *nadis* or Chinese meridians in function—see discussion in Chapter 5) used in traditional massage. These figures were etched into marble tablets, accentuated with black ink, and labeled with verses explaining their content. The tablets—dozens in all—were displayed in two medical

---

34 Griswold (1965), p. 321.
35 Matics (1978), p. 263.

pagodas on the grounds of Wat Pho, surrounded by gardens of rare medicinal herbs from around the kingdom (see Fig. 2).

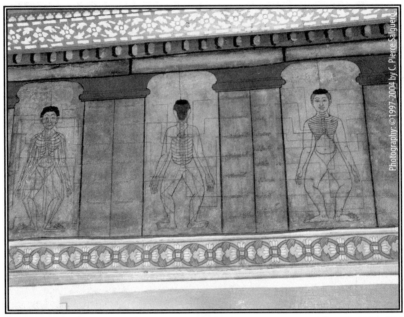

FIG. 2. MASSAGE EPIGRAPHS DEPICT THAI MASSAGE *JAP SEN* POINTS AND *SEN* LINES. MEDICAL PAGODA. WAT PHO, BANGKOK.

Under the direction of the chief physician to the king, Phraya Bamroe Rachabaedya,[36] the extant medical manuscripts and fragments from Ayutthaya were also collected at this time, along with thousands of herbal recipes from physicians across the kingdom.[37] These were compiled and preserved in marble. Displayed alongside the massage diagrams, these tablets included hundreds of recipes dealing with childbirth, pediatrics, and cures for many diseases, including smallpox and tuberculosis.[38] In the words of a contemporary observer, the medical information was presented "in conspicuous and convenient places, so that whosoever will, may freely copy them and treat their diseases accordingly."[39] Prince

36 Apparently at this time, the king's primary physician was Siamese.
37 See Mulholland (1987), p. 13-14 and Matics (1978), p. 254.
38 Matics (1977), p. 146.
39 Bradley (1967), p. 85.

Nivat writes that Rama III envisioned this project as a meritorious act of benevolence to assist his subjects by making them aware of the most efficacious medical texts in the kingdom.[40]

Publication of Medical Texts

Traditional medicine and modern medicine were divided into two separate tracks during the reign of Rama IV (1851-1868), and from this point onwards, TTM was increasingly committed to writing. Mulholland has written a detailed history of the publication of medical texts in the nineteenth and twentieth centuries, and only a summary of these events is repeated here.[41] The authoritative compilation of the royal herbal texts began in 1895, during the reign of Rama V (r. 1868-1910), when by royal decree all known traditional medical manuscripts were copied, compared, and revised by a committee of court doctors at Wat Pho. These manuscripts were used by the first medical school, an institution associated with the Chulalongkorn University (est. 1889) and based at the Sriraj Hospital in Thonburi, across the Chao Phrya River from the capital.

Definitive recensions were drawn up at this time for use by the royal physicians, but the texts were unavailable more widely until 1908, when they were published by Prince Damrong in several compilations: the *Tamra phesat* ("Texts on Medicine"), the *Phaetthayasat songkhro* ("The Study of Medicine"), and an abridged version of the above titles for students, the three-volume *Wetchasu'ksa phaetthayasat sangkhep* ("Manual for Students of Traditional Medicine").[42] The voluminous contents of the *Phaetthayasat songkhro* are outlined in Appendix A at the end of this book.

The mid-twentieth century saw the establishment of the medical college at Wat Pho, and in 1957, the three texts mentioned

---

40 Nivat (1933), p. 143.
41 See Mulholland (1987), Chapter 1.
42 Mulholland (1979a), p. 83.

above were authorized by the Ministry of Public Health to be used by the newly-founded college for the traditional medical curriculum. With the most recent editions published in 1992-93, licensed traditional medicine schools across Thailand continue to utilize these texts as the cornerstone of their training programs today. The Thai Food and Drug Administration also continues to use these texts for the registration of traditional medicines.[43] The Shivagakomarpaj Traditional Medicine Hospital's student manual, excerpts of which are presented in the tables in Chapter 4 and in Appendices B and C, is based on a derivative of this work. Nevertheless, despite their importance to Thai medicine for both practitioners and historians, with the exception of one selection from the *Phaetthayasat songkhro* translated by Mulholland[44] and scattered short quotations in other academic works, these texts have yet to be published in English.

---

43 Chokevivat and Chithaputti (2005), p. 4.
44 Mulholland (1989). I will discuss this text in Chapter 7.

CHAPTER 2

Theravada Buddhism and Medicine in Thailand

Buddhism and Medicine

Thai legend says that the medical system of the *mo boran* was handed down in an unbroken lineage from a handful of sages (Th. *ruesri*, Sk. *rishi*) to modern times via Buddhist texts and oral tradition. The date for the transmission of Buddhism to Southeast Asia from India is given traditionally as the third century B.C.E. At that time the Mauryan king Ashoka is said to have sent two missionaries, Sona and Uttara, from India to Suvnnnabhumi (the "Golden Land," thought to be the modern Burma), where they converted 65,000 people and spread the Buddhist doctrine.[1] The notion that Ashoka ever in fact sent emissaries to Burma has been contested by scholars for many years. G. Coedès states that there is no evidence of Indian culture in Burma before 500 A.D., the date given to fragments of the Pali canon found at Mozaan Mangun.[2] It will be evident from the discussion in the coming chapters that even this time frame is impossible for the introduction of large parts of the Thai medical system. Nevertheless, the arrival of Theravada Buddhism in Southeast Asia brought with it important scriptural traditions of medical knowledge that have had significant impact on medicine. Traditional Thai medicine is usually understood by its practitioners to date from the historical

---

1   Lamotte (1988), p. 293.
2   Coedès (1968), p. 17.

Buddha's lifetime,[3] and this mythology plays a crucial role in unifying the practitioners of Thai medicine today.

Religion has always been one of the major exports of India, and various forms of Buddhism and Hinduism were transmitted from India throughout Asia. The earliest extant form of Buddhism, Theravada ("Teachings of the Elders"), traveled to modern Sri Lanka and Burma, which became Theravada enclaves and remain so to this day. Central Asia, China, and Japan followed a later form of Buddhism, Mahayana ("The Great Vehicle"), while the Khmer regions (modern Cambodia) and the Indonesian islands converted first to Mahayana and then to Hinduism. These areas in some cases adopted India's Brahmanical social system, based on Vedic conceptions of castes and priests, but these institutions were adapted both to suit local conditions as well as to incorporate other influences. Certain areas like Nepal developed a hybrid Buddhist-Hindu tradition centered around Tantric Buddhism (also called Vajrayana, the "Diamond Vehicle"). Other areas, such as the Tibetan kingdoms, seemed to embrace parts of Indian and Chinese culture in a unique synthesis.

The kingdoms in modern-day Thailand were uniquely situated to be on the receiving end of many of these diverse ideas. On the West, they were bordered by the Mon Burmese, a people who had embraced Theravada. On the East, their territory butted against the Khmer Empire, with its unique blend of Hindu and Mahayana influences. Siamese cities also sat along Chinese and Muslim trading routes, and we have already seen Christian missionaries practicing medicine at the Ayutthayan court. It is important to recognize that its strategic geographical location had much influence on the events in Thai history.

Different traditions of Indian religion and medicine arrived in Siam at different times from different sources. Theravada

---

3   As all dates in Indian history are difficult to pin down, the Buddha's lifetime has been the subject of controversy. Scholars had tentatively agreed on the date 486 B.C.E. as a plausible estimate of his death, but recent scholarship has suggested that it may have been even a century later.

Buddhism became the dominant religion in Siam, and Theravada stories would be important narratives for Thai physicians. However, yogic theories originating in Tantric Buddhism and Hinduism (such as vessels, subtle energies, and *hatha-yoga* postures) are also prevalent in Thai medicine. Ayurvedic medicine—related both to Theravada Buddhism as well as yogic practices, but separate from both[4] —also entered Siam at some unknown time.

Ideas coming from different parts of Asia were integrated in Siam, and were blended together with other cultural influences. However, Buddhism and medicine seem to have belonged to different spheres of knowledge and cultural diffusion in Siam, even though these were institutionally related in the elite literate court tradition. Yogic and Ayurvedic knowledge are usually not found among healers outside of the elite literate tradition. In the remoter villages studied by Brun and Schumacher, for example, non-Ayurvedic indigenous T'ai medical ideas predominate.[5] These same villagers, on the other hand, practice Theravada Buddhism, which indicates that Buddhism and medicine did not penetrate all layers of Siamese society hand in hand.

In the Siamese capital, on the other hand, a synthesis developed which tied together T'ai beliefs, Theravada, Ayurveda, and yoga, as well as Chinese and other influences, forming a medical system that became what we know as TTM. Though highly integrated, it is helpful to separate the different influences within this colorful collection of practices, as it assists us greatly in understanding the complexity of TTM. The following chapters therefore will discuss material from the Theravada, Ayurvedic, Yogic, T'ai, Khmer, Chinese, and Western contexts separately, building toward a picture of the integration of these diverse influences.

---

4 Zysk (1993b, 1998) and Wujastyk (2003), p. 260, present detailed arguments for considering these as separate spheres of knowledge.
5 See Brun and Schumacher (1994).

The Buddha's Physician

The principal figure in Thai medical lore is Jivaka Komarabhacca (Th. Shivagakomarpaj or Shivago Komaraphat), claimed by Thai doctors as the founder of their healing tradition. Despite the distinguished place he holds in Thailand, Jivaka is a minor figure in the Pali texts. There are many mentions of him in the canon, including two texts actually named after Jivaka,[6] but even in these, he takes a definitively secondary role to the Buddha and the order of monks. Jivaka is also mentioned as being the owner of a mango grove in Rajagaha, Jivakarama, which he offered for the use of the *sangha* (the community of monks) during their annual rainy-season retreat. Jivaka's skill as a physician and his donation of service to the monastic community is presented in the *Vinaya* as one of the reasons for increasing numbers of ordinations. According to legend, the Buddha has to limit ordination to the healthy in order to prevent abuse of Jivaka's services by the many ill who flocked to the *sangha* to avail of his services.[7]

From virtually all sources, Jivaka seems to have been considered a model healer from the very earliest days of Buddhism.[8] Explicitly medical information in the Pali canon is mostly limited to isolated references to what must have been by then well-known concepts of the body and healing. (There is, for example, mention of the theory of four elements and three *doshas*, philosophical conceptions of the body we will discuss in Part II of this book.[9]) There is one important exception to this generalization, a text in which medical knowledge figures

6   These are two texts called *Jivaka Sutta: Anguttara Nikaya* viii.26, in which Jivaka is given instruction on what it means to be a devoted lay follower, and *Majjhima Nikaya* 55, in which he asks the Buddha about vegetarianism.
7   Demiéville (1985), p. 36.
8   Zysk (1998), p. 147 note 35.
9   See Demiéville (1985) and Zysk (1998) for references to specific passages in the Pali canon discussing these medical ideas.

prominently. The *Mahavagga* section (Chapter 8 of the Pali *Vinaya*), which may be dated to the fourth century B.C.E., presents Jivaka's biography and encounters with patients, providing a wealth of information on contemporary views of healing.[10]

The *Vinaya* is the monastic code, detailing the rules by which the monks must live. The purpose of the Jivaka story in the *Vinaya*, appearing in a section dealing with the types of donations allowable to monastics, is ostensibly to recount the origins of the Buddha's decision to allow the laity to make donations of cloth. Embedded within this seemingly unrelated narrative are several important medical episodes which give us a glimpse of the medical ideal in India in the fourth century B.C.E. That these Jivaka stories became particularly popular among lay Buddhists is indicated by the fact that by the time Buddhism had traveled to China in the first centuries C.E., these passages had been extracted from the *Vinaya*—which was prohibited to the laity—and set out as a separate text to be accessible to all.[11] Two Chinese versions of this text exist today, the *Nainü Qipo Jing* and the *Nainü Qiyu Yinyuan Jing*, in which the protagonist is born with acupuncture needles in his hands. He also uses a magical bough from the "Medicine King" tree to see inside his patients' bodies. In the Tibetan version, he uses a magical gem for this same purpose. I will not refer to the Chinese or Tibetan versions of the Jivaka myths here as it is the Pali text which is canonical in Thailand.

In the Pali, Jivaka's biography begins when the urban council of Rajagaha, inspired by the charms of a courtesan in Vesali, petitions King Bimbisara to install a courtesan of their own. They hire Salavati, with her "utmost beauty of complexion" and "clever dancing, singing and lute playing."[12] This courtesan soon becomes pregnant, however. She delivers in secret, and discards

---

10 See Zysk (1982 and 1998) for details not provided here.
11 Zysk (1998), p. 151 note 9 provides references for the Pali, Chinese and Tibetan sources.
12 *Mahavagga* viii.1.2, trans. Horner (2000), p. 380.

her son in an old winnowing basket on a trash heap, where he lies at the mercy of a flock of crows. The king's son, Prince Abhaya, comes across the baby, and moved by compassion, takes him into his home and names him Jivaka (from *jivati*, or alive) Komarabhacca (apparently from *kaumarabhrtya* meaning "master of the medical science of the treatment of infants").[13]

When Jivaka grows up, he runs away to Taxila, an important town in the Northwest, where he studies with an unnamed medical master for seven years. At the end of this period, he is tested by his teacher, who asks him to find something within a *yojana* (about nine miles) radius that is not medicinal. Jivaka searches the area and proclaims that everything he sees is medicine, and thus passes the test and is given the blessing of his mentor. Jivaka then sets out homeward, but along his way, he stops to heal a merchant's wife, whose family rewards him with 16,000 in cash, two slaves, and a chariot, all of which he presents to his benefactor, Prince Abhaya, upon his return.

Back in Rajagaha and living in the royal palace, Jivaka's fame increases with each client he takes. The *Mahavagga* lists six patients in all. His first is the merchant's wife, whose seven-year-old "incurable disease of the head" is eliminated by one treatment of ghee administered through the nose. The anal fistula of King Bimbisara is then treated successfully with an ointment. Next, in the most dramatic passage of the biography, a merchant of Rajagaha is treated for a fatal disease of the head by trepanation:

> Then Jivaka Komarabhacca, having made the householder, the merchant lie down on a couch, having strapped him to the couch, having cut open the skin of his head, having opened a suture in the skull, having drawn out two living creatures, showed them to the people.[14]

13 Horner (2000), p. 381 note 3. In Thailand his role is principally as the patron saint of children's medicine.
14 Mahavagga viii.1.17, trans. Horner (2000), p. 387.

The son of a merchant of Benares is also dramatically cured of a "twist in the bowels" (caused by "playing at turning somersaults") by slicing his abdomen open, smoothing out the knots, sewing it back up, and applying an ointment. Additionally, King Pajjota of Avanti is cured of a jaundice which "many very great, world-famed doctors had not been able to cure" by a concoction of medicinal ghee surreptitiously administered to the unsuspecting patient. Upon discovering he has been tricked into taking ghee—which he despises—the king flies into a fury and Jivaka flees for his life, only to be later thanked when the king fully recovers.

However, the climax of the biography of Jivaka is the sixth and final episode, a cure administered to the Buddha himself. Jivaka is approached by the Buddha's attendant, Ananda, who tells him that the Buddha has an affliction of the *doshas* of his body (*doshabhisanna*), and that he desires a purgative. Jivaka first tells Ananda to "lubricate" the Buddha's body for several days (probably meaning to ingest oils), after which a mild purgative of medicines mixed with lotuses is administered nasally, causing the Buddha to purge twenty-nine times. After purgation, the patient bathes in hot water, purges a final thirtieth time, and is prescribed a liquid diet of juices until his body returns to normal.

Jivaka in Present-day Thailand

Although the cures attributed to Jivaka do not have much in common with Thai medicine, in Thailand today Jivaka is propitiated as the "Father Doctor" of medicine. The worship of Jivaka involves aspects of orthodox Buddhist and popular religious practice and comprises a major part of the devotional life and identity of the traditional Thai healer. Without exception, every healer I have visited in Thailand has possessed a statue or image of Jivaka, usually seated or standing on an altar alongside an icon of the Buddha, in recognition of his position as the practitioner's primary *khru* (teacher or guru). This has equally been the case for the unlicensed practitioners of non-orthodox forms of healing and for formally-trained physicians and teachers at the authoritative traditional medical schools.

At most Chiang Mai and Bangkok traditional medicine hospitals, schools, and massage clinics, the teachers, students, and patients gather together once or twice a day to recite a prayer to Jivaka in a ceremony of *wai khru*, or "homage to the teacher." Outside the context of medicine, the *wai khru* is a common feature of many Thai arts, and is practiced by shamans, tattoo artists, kick-boxers, and many others who feel that giving the proper thanks to their teachers and lineage is a requirement for success and good luck in their chosen profession. Although more recent teachers may also play a role in the *wai khru* of healers, Jivaka is always an important figure (see Fig. 3).

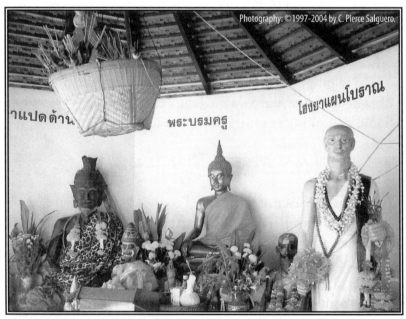

FIG. 3. ALTAR WITH JIVAKA (RIGHT), BUDDHA (CENTER), LUSI (LEFT), AND OTHER MEDICAL AND POPULAR RELIGIOUS FIGURES. SHIVAGAKOMARPAJ TRADITIONAL MEDICINE HOSPITAL, CHIANG MAI.

The *wai khru* ceremony at the Shivagakomarpaj Traditional Medicine Hospital in Chiang Mai takes place in a small pagoda which houses Buddhist icons, statues of Jivaka and other *ruesri*, and ritual paraphernalia typical of Thai temples such as fortune-telling sticks, sacralized water (*nam mon*), and banana leaves folded into elaborate pagoda-like structures (*bai si*). The *wai khru* itself, performed morning and evening at the beginning and end of the workday, is recited in Pali as are all formal Buddhist prayers. It opens with two common Buddhist chants heard at some point during virtually all formal Theravada ceremonies in Thailand. These phrases, chanted in the monotone voice of the Theravada monastic tradition, are the "Homage to the Triple Gem":

> *araham samma sambuddho bhagava, buddham bhaga-vanta abivademi. svakkhato bhagavata dhammo, dham-mam namassami. supatipanno bhagavato savakasangho, sangham namami:* "The Lord, the Perfectly Enlightened and Blessed One—I render homage to the Buddha, the Blessed One. The Teaching so completely explained by him—I bow to the Dhamma. The Blessed One's disciples who have practised well—I bow to the Sangha."[15]

And the "Homage to the Buddha":

> *namo tassa bhagavato arahato samma sambuddhassa:* "Homage to the Blessed, Noble and Perfectly Enlightened One."[16]

These Buddhist phrases are followed by a chant paying homage to Jivaka, which is unknown to the orthodox Theravada tradition outside of the medical field, but draws upon Buddhist language, imagery, and stock phrases. This chant is found in

15 Translation by Saddhatissa and Walshe (1994), p. 3.
16 Translation by Saddhatissa and Walshe (1994), p. 3.

various forms throughout Chiang Mai and Bangkok, but invariably lauds Jivaka as a moral follower of the precepts, and is replete with praise of the Buddha. The following stanza appears at the beginning of every version of this recitation I have seen:

om namo shivago sirasa ahang karuniko sapasatanang osata tipamantang papaso suriyajantang komarapato pagasesi wantami bandito sumetaso aloka sumanhomi:[17] "Homage to you Jivaka, I bow down. You are kind to all beings and bring to all beings divine medicine, and shine light like the sun and moon. I worship he who releases sickness, wise and enlightened Komarabaccha. May I be healthy and happy."[18]

The *wai khru* at the Shivagakomarpaj Hospital continues:

piyo-tewa manusanang piyo-proma namutamo piyo-naka supananang pinisriyong namamihang namoputaya navon-navean nasatit-nasatean a-himama navean-nave napitang-vean naveanmahako a-himama piyongmama namoputaya na-a nava loka payati winasanti: "He is beneficent to gods and human beings, beneficent to Brahma. I pay homage to the great one. He is beneficent to *naga* and *supanna*.... I pay homage. Homage to the Buddha.... Honor to the Buddha. May all diseases be released."[19]

The *wai khru* ceremony thus uses formal Buddhist rites and Theravada imagery to honor a figure from the Pali canon, reaffirming the central role of Buddhist faith and lore in the

---

17 Source: Chaichakan (1997), frontispiece.
18 Based on translation by W.Y. Bandara, personal communication.
19 Based on translation by W.Y. Bandara, personal communication. Ellipses indicate words that remain untranslated. Brahma, in Theravada mythology, though not an eternal god, is the highest *thewada*, or celestial reincarnation, and *nagas* and *supanna* are mythical earth-beings. The implication here is that Jivaka is beneficent to all levels of beings, high and low, throughout the universe.

practice of Thai medicine. The *wai khru* is not the only example of the integration of Jivaka into everyday life. A Jivaka icon is often placed in prominent locations for temple-goers to worship, for example presiding over the main entrance to the national temple, Wat Phra Kaew (see Fig. 4). When visiting a traditional hospital such as Shivagakomarpaj, it is customary to visit the pagoda housing the Jivaka statues and pay homage upon entering and leaving the facility before an altar that contains statues of Buddhas as well as famous *ruesri* or medical sages (the altar in Fig. 3 is from Shivagakomarpaj's main shrine).

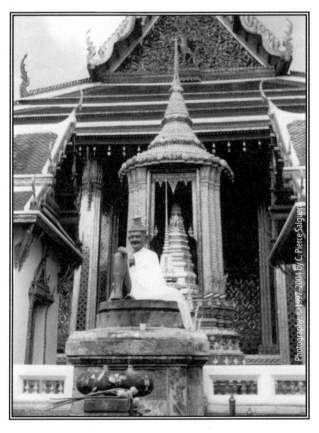

FIG. 4. JIVAKA PRESIDING OVER THE ENTRANCE TO THE NATIONAL TEMPLE. WAT PHRA KAEW, BANGKOK.

Jivaka, then, is an important figure for not only doctors, but patients as well. In fact, one of the main teachings of the traditional medical school at the Shivagakomarpaj Hospital is that religious practice (Th. *chittanamai*)—and by this it is invariably meant Theravada Buddhist meditation and ritual—is one of the major disciplines of Thai medicine, alongside herbalism/dietary regimen and massage/acupressure. The "three branches of Thai medicine," as they are called at Shivagakomarpaj, are represented in the architecture of the facility itself, which houses a medical school in the north wing, an herbal dispensary and massage clinic to the south, and a pagoda containing the main shrine to the Buddha and Jivaka centrally located on the premises. The very placement of the shrine at the midpoint of the complex points to a self-consciousness about the centrality of Buddhist religion and the "Father Doctor" Jivaka in the practice of traditional medicine.[20]

Buddhist Philosophy and TTM

Theravada Buddhism had been the dominant religious tradition in Siam since the founding of Sukothai, and it is therefore no surprise that efforts would be made by physicians to legitimize traditional medical practice through association with Jivaka, the Buddha's physician in the Pali scriptures. So, it is not unexpected to find practitioners of the medical arts propitiating the "Father Doctor" or including Buddhist ritual in their healing practices.

In fact, however, Buddhism is not only a legitimizing force in theory, but a relevant part of the practice of TTM. Even today, Buddhism continues to play a central role in the delivery of traditional medicine. It has already been noted that the most important medical artifacts of the Bangkok era are housed

---

20 This was the layout of the hospital when I left in 2001. I understand it has been renovated since that time and that the layout has changed.

in Wat Pho, a prominent temple which continues to be the spiritual center for TTM nationwide. Likewise, on a regional level, many temples are known for medical libraries and monks often serve as community medical practitioners. Monks have for some time now been co-opted into the national plan for healthcare, and trained to deliver primary care, particularly in poorer areas.[21] For the most part, monks have had a positive view toward their role as curers, this despite the fact that the monastic code (the *Vinaya*) explicitly prohibits monks from administering medicine to laypeople, and some texts even label medicine a "base and wrong means of livelihood."[22]

Another example of the contemporary integration of Buddhism and medicine is seen in the inclusion into the TTM framework of "the application of Buddhism or rites and rituals for mental health care."[23] The practice of *dhammanamai*, or the "holistic care of the body, the mind, the society, and the environment," forwards a platform of health based on Buddhist relaxation techniques and morality.[24] For the most part, these practices draw from popular religion and not from canonical texts, allowing a greater amount of flexibility in incorporating non-Buddhist techniques such as proper diet and *ruesri dat ton* (the traditional stretching exercises outlined in Chapter 1). This fusion of healing with Buddhist philosophy serves as a unifying force to legitimize diverse practices from many sources, and also places medical knowledge under the umbrella of a common religious tradition. One of the themes of the last chapter of this book will be the ways in which Thai practitioners use Buddhism to unify a range of practices imported from a diversity of sources in order to construct modern TTM.

21 See Gosling (1985) for information in this paragraph.
22 *Digha Nikaya* i.11. Cited in Demiéville (1995), p. 36.
23 Chokevivat (2005), p. 4.
24 Chokevivat and Chithapatti (2005), p. 16-18.

CHAPTER 3

Eclectic Influences on Thai Culture & Medicine

Khmer Influence

The Khmer Empire—which ruled over most of modern-day Cambodia from the ninth to the thirteenth centuries C.E.— controlled at times a large region of Southeast Asia and was one of the major cultural and political forces in the region. Based at the capital, Angkor, the empire extended its power and influence into parts of modern-day Cambodia, Laos, Vietnam, and Thailand. The Khmer court was marked by its own species of Brahmanism imported from India. This system featured a caste hierarchy headed by Brahmans, as well as rituals based on the Vedas. As shown by the colossal ruins of Angkor Wat, Hinduism as well as Mahayana Buddhism (a later form of Buddhism that developed in the Common Era) were also major factors in Khmer culture.

Chapter 1 mentioned how early Siamese kingdoms came in continual contact with Khmer culture. Historians have remarked that, in the seventeenth-century, Ayutthaya exhibited many similarities with Angkorian society, government, and ritual.[1] Other historians have pointed out that many similarities persist between modern Thai political institutions—particularly royal ceremonies—and their Khmer antecedents.[2]

---

1 Griswold and Nagara (1975), p. 69.
2 See Wales (1977).

Khmer influence can be seen in many Thai folk practices today as well, and the role that Khmer symbolism and imagery continues to play in Thai healing is significant. There is some cause for speculation that the transmission to Siam of much of its Ayurvedic medical material occurred through the Khmer regions. Until recently, most Siamese medical texts (like religious texts) were written on palm leaf manuscripts in the Pali language using the Khmer script (*khom*). It was only in the Bangkok period that the Thai script began to be used to write herbal texts. The organization of Khmer herbal manuscripts is identical to that of typical Thai herbal manuscripts and is based, like many Thai texts, on the four element theory.[3] There are similarities in content as well as structure, indicating a shared pharmacopoeia between India, the Khmer Empire, and Siam. Much more research is needed to delineate the similarities between the medical practices of the Khmer and Siamese.

Chinese Influence

Another source of much influence on Thai medicine throughout history is the huge Chinese population that has been present in Southeast Asia for centuries. Many historical and cultural connections between Chinese and Thai culture exist, a fact that should not surprise us given Thailand's geographical location and the reach of the powerful Chinese empires' influence throughout the region. Contact between these groups was continuous throughout the history of both. As discussed in Chapter 1, the origins of the T'ai people can be traced to the coast of modern-day Vietnam, on the

---

3   Chhem (2004), p. 34-35. A cursory glance at the pharmacopoeia presented in a Khmer manuscript translated by Chhem, entitled "The Treatment of the Four Diseases," confirms links with both Indian and Thai medicine.

southern border of Tang China (dynastic dates 618-907). As the T'ais migrated out of this homeland in the eighth through the twelfth centuries, they constantly interacted with the expanding Chinese empire and even settled in the southern region of modern-day Yunnan Province. (To this day, this region is known in Chinese as Xishuangbanna, a Sinified pronunciation of Sipsongpanna, which is Thai for "twelve thousand rice districts.") The Dai, a Chinese minority group of T'ai descent which populates this area today, share certain ceremonies, language, and other aspects of culture with other T'ai groups.[4]

Not only were there T'ais in China, but there were Chinese in Siam as well. The Chinese were a mobile, mercantile population, intent on trade and colonization. Some scholars believe that Chinese presence in Southeast Asian commercial centers predated the arrival of the T'ais themselves.[5] Certainly, they maintained constant presence in Southeast Asia throughout most of the last millennium. Chinese influence is reflected in Sukothai pottery styles, among the earliest cultural artifacts from Siam.[6] By the Ayutthaya period the Chinese population in the city is known to have included merchants, traders, scholars, artisans, actors, pig-breeders, and notably, physicians.[7] Many features of what we know today as Traditional Chinese Medicine (TCM) were already well developed in China by the Song Dynasty (960-1280). Thus practices such as cautery (or moxibustion), acupuncture, massage, and herbal medicine would without doubt have been known to Chinese doctors in Siam. Chinese medicine was apparently well received in Ayutthaya: we have already noted the fact that de la Loubère numbers Chinese physicians among the king's retinue.

---

4   See Terwiel (1978b).
5   Skinner (1957), p. 1.
6   Tarling (1992), p. 169.
7   Skinner (1957), p. 15.

In the nineteenth century, Daniel Beach Bradley observed in his papers several Siamese recipes, such as the following, which bear a strikingly Chinese stamp:

> One portion of rhinosceros [sic] horn, one portion of elephant's tusk, one of tyger's [sic], and the same of croc-odile's teeth; one of bear's teeth, one portion composed of three parts bones of vulture, raven, and goose; one portion of bison and another of stag's horn; one portion of sandal.[8]

With the inclusion of so many exotic animal parts—a prac-tice not typically found in Ayurveda—it is likely that recipes like these are examples of Chinese medicine in Siam in the nineteenth century.

On the whole, the story of Chinese immigration in Thailand has been both a peaceful and a mutually beneficial process for both ethnic groups. Despite the fact that Chinese populations in neighboring Malaysia and Indonesia have suffered politi-cal and social persecutions at various points in the twentieth century, the Thai-Chinese have been considered to be a model for successful integration of overseas Chinese into Southeast Asian cultures.[9] Today, Chinese immigrants make up over ten percent of the population of Thailand, and control an even larger proportion of the economic resources of the country. Most of this Chinese immigrant population has come from Guangdong Province in Southeast China, but historically significant minorities also include Hainanese, Cantonese, Hakka, Hokkien, and more recently, Yunnanese.[10] Chinese communities and temples are a visible feature of a Thai city of any size, and their religious events play a central role in the

---

8   Bradley (1967), p. 86.
9   See Kenjiro (1967).
10 Formoso (1996), p. 219 and Hill (1992), p. 315.

Thai festival calendar. Often, these functions are as important to the Thai majority as their own festivals. (We will explore one such ceremony in Chapter 7.)

Today, Chinese influence continues within the orthodox Thai herbal tradition. TCM is recognized as one of the three official medical traditions by the central government, and Chinese doctors are quite visible in Thai cities. In 1988, Van Esterik wrote that most pharmacies in Bangkok were owned by Chinese proprietors, and that Chinese medicines were sold at all but "a very few" of the city's pharmacies.[11] Though I have not been able to find hard data, my impression is that Chinese physicians outnumber *mo boran* by a considerable margin, particularly in large urban centers with affluent Chinese populations like Bangkok and Chiang Mai. Chinese pharmacies, acupuncturists, and massage clinics are encountered both within Chinese and Thai neighborhoods.

Even in the clinics and hospitals staffed by Thais that I visited in the late 1990s and early 2000s, Chinese remedies were commonplace. Well-known Chinese herbs, such as ginseng (*Panax ginseng*), are today found at virtually all Thai herbal shops, as well as in many grocery stores and corner markets across Thailand. Furthermore, I have also seen many Thai herbalists utilize Chinese diagnostics such as analysis of the irises, tongue, and pulse in their herbal practices. Likewise, some Chinese remedies appear in the training manuals of the Shivagakomarpaj Hospital (see Appendices B and C), indicating that the medicinal use of these substances is taught as part of the *mo boran* curriculum.

Despite the role Chinese medicine plays in Thailand today, however, it is not well represented in the literature or textbooks of TTM schools. On the whole, modern medical texts prioritize the Indian system—its terminology, pharmacology, and theoretical structure—over both indigenous Thai practices

---

11 Van Esterik (1988), p 753. I am unaware of any updates to this statistic.

and other foreign influence. I will explore reasons for this in the final chapter of this book.

Western Influence

As in many areas of the non-Western world, European medicine was first introduced to Siam by Christian missionaries. The first Jesuit hospital was established at Ayutthaya in 1676. By the nineteenth century, an American missionary doctor, Daniel Beech Bradley, served as the king's physician.[12] "Mo Bradley" introduced smallpox inoculation, and provided training in this technique to the court physicians. The first government medical school, Sriraj, opened in 1889 in Bangkok, and taught Western biomedical science alongside traditional herbalism.[13] Public health institutions were established throughout the late nineteenth and early twentieth centuries.[14]

Public health and medicine were among the most powerful tools of Western colonialism. Historically, a feature of European colonialism and Western-influenced modernization has been the denigration of traditional medical knowledge as "superstitious" and "backward." The two most well-known examples of Asian medical tradition, Indian Ayurveda and Traditional Chinese Medicine, both suffered times of repression and competition by Western biomedicine during which the indigenous living tradition was severely threatened. Although traditional doctors still practiced throughout the period, these two traditions were fully resurrected as respectable healing systems only in the second half of the twentieth century as a part of broader anti-Western nationalist movements.

With the exception of a short period of Japanese occupation in World War II, Thailand ("Land of the Free") never

---

12 See Lord (1969).
13 Van Estrik (1988), p. 755.
14 See Wibulbolprasert (2005), Chatper 1, for an outline of the history of public health.

experienced an era of colonial domination, and thus a different dynamic obtained. However, traditional Thai institutions suffered a marked loss of prestige in the nineteenth and twentieth centuries with the increasing presence of Western medicine. Since the introduction of biomedicine, the Thai government has oscillated between support, benign neglect, and repression of native traditions.

The twentieth century was a period of mixed success for TTM. For the first part of the century, the government sidelined traditional medicine in favor of biomedicine. For example, laws in 1923 and 1936 outlawed the majority of TTM practitioners within the health service system. It was not until a 1978 declaration of the WHO supporting traditional medicine worldwide for primary healthcare in developing countries that the Ministry of Public Health began to unambiguously promote the practice of traditional medicine. Since 1978, TTM has received increasing levels of support from the government. This process will be discussed in the last chapter of this book.

Thai medicine continues to interact with Western influences. Medical policy plays a significant role in post-colonial globalization, as Western governments, NGOs, corporations, and organizations like the WHO continue to intervene in Thai medical affairs (most recently, for example, in the bird-flu outbreak), and continue to exert an influence on Thai institutions. In traditional medicine, the presence of large numbers of Western tourists who are becoming patients and students in Bangkok and Chiang Mai Thai massage clinics and schools can not but influence the way in which this knowledge is taught and practiced.

A trend toward integrative medicine has taken hold in Thailand. A statistic cited at the beginning of this book demonstrates that the vast majority of Thailand's biomedical institutions incorporate TTM to some extent. On the other side of the divide, some universities have recently begun Master's programs which build on the traditional three-year TTM training with additional biomedical training, and thus continue to blur the lines between Thai and Western medicine.

Certain aspects of biomedical practice have been appropriated and put to use by non-elite and untrained healers in culturally unique ways. For example, I have heard reports of "injection doctors," who tour the Thai countryside administering injections of antibiotics, other drugs, or even placebos, to their patients at certain points on the body with magic or ritual significance. This is simply one among many examples of how biomedical ideas are not necessarily always understood or implemented in the way Western organizations intend. Thai communities continue to accept and modify the cultural influences they come in contact with, and this continues to be a highly localized process.

The fact that these two systems, TTM and biomedicine, are both officially recognized by the government today does not mean that they are always perceived as being equals by patients. Studies of how patients make decisions about healthcare, how they choose between different types of practitioners, and how they negotiate the diversity in the "medical marketplace" would be most welcomed additions to the field.

Other Influences

Because they seem to play less of a formative role in TTM, and because it is impossible to discuss all aspects of medicine in Thailand in a book of this size, I will not dwell on the influences listed in this final section. I will simply point out the existence of many more eclectic cultural and social forces on medicine that await analysis and research.

It is not known to what extent Islamic medical influence has been a factor in the historical development of TTM, but it does remain a factor in contemporary practice. The southern part of modern Thailand is populated by a Muslim majority, who practice very different forms of healing based on Arabic and Malay medical traditions.[15] According to Golomb, significant borrowing routinely takes place between Malay and Thai groups in these areas, and he reports that sorcerers of minority ethnicity are often sought out by Thai patients as ritual specialists in curative magic.[16]

Other regional ethnic differences also await future research by scholars. Six distinct Hill Tribes, including the Karen, Hmong, Lahu, Akha, Lisu, Yao, and Lawa, as well as significant Burmese and Lao immigrants, populate the north of Thailand. The contributions of these groups to Thai medical culture has remained largely unevaluated, but in certain places (such as at the Shivagakomarpaj Traditional Medicine Hospital, which claims to incorporate Hill-Tribe medical knowledge) appear to play significant roles. The same could be said of the ethnically Thai people from remote regions of the country. Isaan, for example, the under-developed northeastern part of Thailand, is well-known around Chiang Mai for its potent magicians and healers. Whether this reputation has to do with a feature of Isaan medicine, or of Chiang Mai's stereotyping of that region, would be an interesting study.

---

15 See discussions of southern Thai healing in Golomb (1985).
16 Golomb (1985), p. 194-201.

PART II

Traditional Thai Medicine

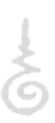

CHAPTER 4

A Thai Ayurveda

The few hints that remain of the medicine of the Ayutthayan court do not give the impression that Siamese medicine was dominated by Indian thought. In contrast, the Thai medical tradition enshrined at Wat Pho in the nineteenth century and taught today across the country draws heavily and self-consciously from Ayurveda and *hatha-yoga*. The next two chapters will show that TTM today continues to draw heavily on Ayurvedic and yogic views of the body and of healing.

In these two chapters, I will draw upon my experiences training as a practitioner at the Shivagakomarpaj Traditional Medicine Hospital in Chiang Mai, Thailand, from 1997-2001. Founded in 1973 by the *mo boran* Sintorn Chaichakan (who trained at the Wat Pho medical school), Shivagakomarpaj has become one of the most prestigious traditional medical training centers in Northern Thailand. The institution today operates both a TTM hospital with in-patient facilities and a medical school which prepares students to sit for the national Ministry of Public Health examination.

It is dangerous to make generalizations about traditional Thai medicine from the observation of just one school. In the absence of full standardization, schools across Thailand offer quite different curricula and experiences for students. Moreover, Shivagakomarpaj is unique in that the school's founder incorporated local northern Thai knowledge and Hill-Tribe traditions into the training program. However, because Shivagakomarpaj prepares students for the national exam, it can in broad outline be considered to be a representative example of an institution within the TTM tradition.

Indian Ayurveda

The term Ayurveda ("the science of life" or "the science of longevity") was first used to refer to medicine in the *Mahabharata*,[1] an epic text that was compiled over the first half of the first millennium B.C.E.[2] The fundamental texts of Ayurveda are the *Caraka Samhita* (parts of which date as early as the third century B.C.E.) and the *Sushruta Samhita* (as early as the last few centuries B.C.E.).[3]

Historians of Indian medicine believe that the ideas described within these texts grew out of medical traditions shared among early Buddhists, Upanishadic philosophers, and other wandering ascetics known collectively in Sanskrit as *sramana*.[4] The *Caraka* and *Sushruta* share much material with the Jivaka stories in the *Vinaya* and other sections of the Pali canon, in particular a rational approach to healing, similarities in medical therapies, and a variety of shared herbal compounds. Likewise, the Ayurvedic *samhitas* share with the *Vinaya's* medicine a model by which health is seen as a continual struggle to balance internal and external forces: environment, diet, morality, exercise, and other aspects of daily regimen play a central role in the Ayurvedic outlook. The *samhitas* are also based on the theories of *mahabhutas* (or proto-elements) and *doshas* (or humors), which appear for the first time in Pali Buddhist texts.

The *Caraka* and *Sushruta* have, more than any other texts, defined the classical Ayurvedic tradition, but these were not the final word in Ayurveda. Many more treatises would be produced,

1 Wujastyk (2003), p. 394.
2 Flood (1996), p. 105.
3 Exact dating of these texts has been controversial. In this book, I follow Wujastyk (2003).
4 See Zysk (1998), Chapter 2, for information in this paragraph.

reflecting changes in theory and practice, and the practice is still redefining itself continually today.[5] Later influences, beyond the scope of this chapter, included Persian alchemy in the medieval period, Western public health brought by colonists in the early modern period, as well as influence from biomedicine in the nineteenth and twentieth centuries—not to mention the recent trend of "New Age Ayurveda" as exemplified by individuals such as Vasant Lad and Deepak Chopra.[6] However, these two texts, established in their current form by 500 C.E., have remained the two most central works in the Ayurvedic tradition. These classical medical writings circulated widely throughout South and Southeast Asia wherever Indian culture traveled, and deeply influenced medical practices throughout this region, particularly in Thailand.

Thai Ayurveda

Modern TTM, like Ayurvedic medicine, is based on the idea that health and disease are largely internal processes. In both systems, the balance of four proto-elements (Th. *that*) is considered of utmost importance to optimal health and longevity. In Thai etiology, the elements can be upset through climate change, food intake, emotional or psychological factors, heredity, allergic reactions, environmental factors, astrological forces, and sorcery, among other influences, and they can be therapeutically manipulated through the use of dietary regimes or medicinal herbs.[7] The elements are the "foundation of the whole body and the foundation of life and durability," and they provide the critical link between symptoms and treatment.[8]

---

5 See Wujastyk (2003) for selections from major Ayurvedic texts in translation.
6 See Zysk (2001) for critique of this movement.
7 Ratarasarn (1989), Chapter 2, discusses these disease etiologies extensively.
8 Ratarasarn (1989), p. 62-63. See her Chapter 1 for a detailed discussion of diseases associated with each element.

Like in the Ayurvedic literature, Thai medical texts break down the world into categories based on the predominant element(s) present in any substance or phenomenon. For example, the earth element, with the quality of solidity, relates to all solid objects in nature, such as rocks and wood. The water element, with the quality of fluidity, relates to all that is liquid. The air element, with the quality of movement, relates to that which is moving and flexible, such as the wind. The fire element, with the quality of heat, relates to hot and cold temperatures. Like in Ayurveda, in some Thai texts, a fifth element, ether, represents the void or the absence of the other four. The elements and their qualities are outlined in Table 4.1.

TABLE 4.1. THE ELEMENTS (*THAT*)

Element	Quality	Examples
Earth (*Th. din*)	Solid	Rocks, metals
Water (*Th. nam*)	Liquid	Water, fruits
Air (*Th. lom*)	Movement	Wind, weather, time
Fire (*Th. fai*)	Heat	Sun, summer heat, fire
Ether (*Th. akat*)	Void, emptiness	Spaces, holes, voids

This elemental model provides the *mo boran* with the necessary theoretical tools to analyze his patients' symptoms and draw conclusions about both cause and treatment. Like the rest of the phenomenal world, Thai texts classify parts of the human body by their relation to one of the primordial elements, based on the perception of the predominance of one quality or another. For example, blood, predominating in the quality of liquidity, would be classified as a water-element body-part, while more solid bones would be intuitively categorized under earth. A traditional list of fifty-two body parts categorized by element appears in Table 4.2. This list is exceedingly similar to lists found both in Theravada Buddhist texts as well as the Ayurvedic *samhitas*.[9]

TABLE 4.2. THE ELEMENTS AND THE PARTS OF THE HUMAN BODY[10]

Earth (20)
Hair, body hair, nails, teeth, skin, flesh, tendons, bones, marrow, spleen, heart, liver, fascia, kidneys, lungs, large intestine, small intestine, undigested food, waste matter, brain

Water (12)
Bile, mucus, pus, blood, perspiration, body fat, tears, lymph, saliva, clear mucus, fluid in the joints, urine

Air (6)
Air which starts at the feet and rises to the head, air which starts from the head and descends to the feet, air in the abdominal cavity, air which circulates in the intestines and stomach, air which circulates throughout the body, the breath inhaled and exhaled

Fire (4)
Body heat which warms the body, body heat which makes the body feel hot and uncomfortable, heat which causes senility and causes the body to wither and dry, the heat to digest food

Ether (10)[11]
Two eyes, two nostrils, the two ears, the mouth, anus, urethra, vagina or seminal passage

---

9 For example, compare *Mahasatipatthana Sutta* (*Digha Nikaya* ii.293) and Chapter seven of the *Sharira Sthana* of the *Caraka Samhita*.
10 Source: Abridged from Mulholland (1979a), pp. 90-95, except Ether (see next note).
11 Ether's body parts are not always included in lists like this one, and are missing from Mulholland's list although present in the Shivagakomarpaj materials. The body parts associated with this element are the body's orifices.

The *mo boran* diagnoses the cause of disease through the practice of *that chao ruan*, or identification of the elemental imbalance. Imbalance can be due to either excess or depletion, and the physician will be able to recognize the signs of either of these conditions by the patient's symptoms. If a patient exhibits a characteristic that correlates with one of the above body parts or processes, the diagnosis is relatively straightforward. For example, the retention of fluid can be interpreted as an excess of the water element, or a drop in body heat can be depletion of fire element.

These diagnostic considerations would be amplified by analysis of the elements in the individual patient's environment, as well as in the constitution. For example, the hot season tends to agitate the fire element, so those conceived in or born in summer may have natural tendencies toward imbalance of fire, and everyone should be more cautious about keeping the fire in balance during this season. Excess of fire can be managed through eating cooling foods, drinks and herbs, while depletion of fire can be managed through eating heating substances. Astrological diagnosis as well as physical examination of heart rate, pulse, temperature, palpation, and so forth, may also be used.[12]

As in the Indian system, the Thai elements are manifested in the human body in the form of three humors. The Thai *doshas* correlate exactly with the classical Ayurvedic (see Table 4.3). The first, called *di* in Thai, meaning bile, correlates to the fire element. *Lom*, or wind, correlates to air. Finally, *salet*, or mucus, correlates to the water element. As in Indian Ayurveda, the earth and ether elements are not generally seen as being responsible for disease, but when the imbalance of other *doshas* corrupts the earth element, the disease is considered incurable.[13] In both systems, the *doshas* are thought to be fluids which circulate

---

12 Chokevivat and Chuthaputti (2005), p. 3.
13 Compare Mulholland (1979b), p. 30, and Demiéville (1985), p. 67.

throughout the body's many vessels, and when they are affected by the elemental imbalance, they cause disease.

TABLE 4.3. THE THREE HUMORS (*DOSHA*)

Thai *Dosha*	Ayurvedic Equivalent	Associated Element	Properties/ Symptoms	Example Diseases
Di	*Pitta*	Fire	Bile, anger, heat	Fevers, infections
Lom	*Vata*	Air	Movement, agitation	Aging, debility
Salet	*Slesma*	Water	Mucus, lethargy	Congestion, lethargy

Thai Herbal Prescription

Thai medicine utilizes a system of classification of pharmacological substances by flavor which provides the fundamental connection between specific symptoms and the prescription of herbal remedies. These flavor categories are similar to those that are used in the prescriptive theory of classical Ayurvedic sources. The Ayurvedic tradition established in the *Caraka Samhita* maintains six flavors. The Thai tradition maintains various flavor systems, but these lists nevertheless are exceedingly similar (see Table 4.4). Although there are other schemes, the nine-taste system predominates in the Shivagakomarpaj texts. A tenth Thai flavor, bland, is included in these texts, but is not usually counted as a tenth flavor, as it represents a lack of the other flavors. (This is comparable to the ether element, which represents a void or lack of the other elements.)

Each flavor has a known effect of raising or lowering the excess or depletion of specific elements. Thus, when the *mo*

TABLE 4.4. FLAVOR SYSTEMS COMPARED

Flavor:	Bitter (khom)	Sour (priao)	Sweet (wan)	Pungent (phet ron)	Salty (khem)	Astringent (fat)	Aromatic (hom yen)	Oily (man)	Toxic[14] (mao-buea)
Ayurvedic system:	X	X	X	X	X	X			
Thai systems:									
4 Flavors		X		X	X	X			
6 Flavors	X	X	X	X	X	X			
8 Flavors	X	X	X	X	X	X	X	X	
9 Flavors	X	X	X	X	X	X	X	X	X

boran has successfully identified the elemental imbalance causing a disease, the step from this to a prescription is theoreti-
cally straightforward. For example, Table 4.5, a selection from
the Shivagakomarpaj student manual, lists the elements, the
correlating flavors, associated diseases, and the main herbal
medicines for each category.

TABLE 4.5. FLAVORS AND ELEMENTS IN TTM[15]

The Four Elements and their Associated Flavors:

Element	Flavors	Main Herbal Treatments
Earth	Astringent, sweet, oily, salty	*Piper sylvaticum*
Water	Sour, bitter, toxic	*Piper sarmentosum* [Wild pepper]
Air	Hot	*Piper ribesoides* Wall [Sakahn]
Fire	Aromatic, bland	*Plumbago zelyanica* Linn (root) [Plumbago]
Ether	N/A	*Zingiber officinal* [Ginger]

14 This term is translated by Mulholland (1979a, p. 86) as "poisonous, intoxicating, and/or addic-
tive," and according to her, "normally refers to drugs which act on the central nervous system."
15 Chaichakan (1997). Sections of the current Shivagakomarpaj's manual for students of Thai
Medicine were translated in 1997 by a translation team in Chiang Mai, Thailand, that included
the author, Pikul Termyod, and Tananan Willson. The original material is in tabular format,
which I have preserved, although I have replaced column headings with my own. Brackets []
indicate common English name (Thai used when English is unknown or non-existent).

The Nine Flavors (plus Bland):

Flavor	Indications	Examples
Astringent	Liver, digestion	*Tamarindus indica* [Tamarind] bark, *Andrographis paniculata* [Chiretta]
Sweet	Energy	*Saccharum spp.* [Sugar cane], melon, honey
Toxic	Parasites	*Datura metel* [Datura], *Papaver somniferum* [Opium]
Bitter	Lungs, fever	*Tinospora tuberculata* Beumee [Heart-leaved moonseed]
Pungent/Hot	Colds	*Capsicum spp.* [peppers], *Aegle marmelos* [Bengal quince], *Acorus calamus Linn.* [Calamus], *Syzygium aromaticum* [Cloves], *Ocymum sanctum* [Holy basil]
Oily/Nutty	Energy, joints, muscle	*Nelumbo nucifera* [Lotus] seed, nuts, *Castanospormum australe* [Black beans], *Artocarpus integrifolia* [Jackfruit] seed, *Tamarindus indica* [Tamarind] seed

The Nine Flavors (plus Bland): *(continued)*		
Flavor	Indications	Examples
Aromatic	Heart, "bad blood"	*Nelumbo nucifera* [Lotus] and *Jasminum spp.* [Jasmine] flowers, powdered and eaten.
Salty	Constipation, gas	Salt, seafood
Sour	Fever, "bad blood"	*Citrus aurantifolia* [Lime], *Citrus hystix* [Kaffir lime], *Tamarindus indica* [Tamarind] fruit, *Mangifera indica* [Mango], *Ananas cososus* [Pineapple]
Bland (absence of other nine)	Poisoning, chronic thirst	White vegetables, *Cucurbita spp.* [Pumpkin]

In practice, herbal simples (single medicinal herbs) such as those listed in Table 4.5 are hardly ever used. Most herbalists prescribe compounds formulated with dozens of ingredients, measured out in specific ratios. These recipes may combine herbs from many—if not all—flavor categories in different proportions. Thai herbs are often compounded in combinations familiar to Indian Ayurveda. The famous Ayurvedic recipe for Triphala (*Terminalia belerica*, *Terminalia chebula*, and *Phyllanthus emblica*), for example, is frequently found in Thai medical manuscripts.[16]

16 Mulholland (1979b), p. 35.

Another very important Thai medical prescription is the "family of five," five herbs frequently found together in varying proportions. A typical recipe for a "family of five" compound is found below, quoted from Wat Pho's 1969 *Manual for Studies in Thai Pharmacy*:

When the elements are defective, and cause discolored stools—like black, red, white, or green—use "the family of five" in the following way:

+ 4 units of leaf, flower, and root of *Plumbago zelyanica*, respectively
+ 6 units of leaf, flower, and root of *Piper aff. boehmeriaefolium*, respectively
+ 10 units of leaf, flower, and root of *Zingiber officinale*, respectively
+ 12 units of leaf, flower, and root of *Piper sarmentosum*, respectively
+ 20 units of leaf, flower, and root of *Piper sylvaticum*, respectively[17]

When looking at the extensive lists of medicinal substances used in TTM, many parallels to Ayurveda are apparent despite the quite different flora and fauna found in India and Thailand. Appendix B and Appendix C, for example, which are excerpted from the Shivagakomarpaj manuals, list dozens of Thai medicines categorized both by symptom and flavor category. Among the many specific plants named, over 80 percent are either themselves also found, or share a genus with plants also found, in the classical Ayurvedic pharmacopoeia.[18] The other 20 percent consists of popular Chinese remedies and indigenous plants with no Ayurvedic or Chinese counterpart. Of the 80 percent,

---

17 Brun & Schumacher (1994), p. 15.
18 I used the *Madanapalanighantu*, a major pharmacopoeia from 14th-century India (Dash 1991), for this comparison.

moreover, not only are the individual herbal substances similar, but they are in both systems categorized quite similarly. (A hot flavor herb, for example, is typically labeled as such by both traditions.)

Judging from this one sample of Thai medicine, the parallels with Indian herbalism are striking. Of course, in this comparison, I am using a single Thai and a single Ayurvedic source, and the teachings of a single Thai medical school. However, as the material translated in the appendices was excerpted by Sintorn Chaichakan of the Shivagakomarpaj school from the Ministry of Public Health's *Tumea Phadphanboran Tuapai, Saka Vedhakram* and *Saka Phesadhakram*—texts used across Thailand to prepare students for the national examination—we can infer that the contents give a representative sampling of the pharmacopoeia current among modern *mo boran* with formal training. A full catalog of the traditional Thai pharmacopoeia is lacking in the academic literature, and thus any comprehensive comparative work on Thai and Indian Ayurvedic prescriptions is wanting. More research is needed, but I believe we can generalize that modern Thai medicine as taught by the authoritative schools today is closely analogous to the Ayurvedic *samhitas* in etiology, prescriptive theory, and therapeutic substances.

CHAPTER 5

A Thai Yoga

If we find the connection with Indian tradition to be evident when it comes to Thai herbal medicine, it is similarly the case with Thai therapeutic massage (Th. *nuad boran*). We have already seen that a dearth of historical materials hinders the study of the history of Thai medicine, and nowhere is this more apparent than in the study of traditional massage. While there are very few historical sources on Thai herbal medicine, there are none of which I am aware that discuss massage in any detail prior to the production of the tablets at Wat Pho. Unfortunately, despite the popularity of Thai massage in the past decade or two both in Thailand and among Western enthusiasts, these tablets themselves remain untranslated and unstudied in detail. However, through comparative study of contemporary practice, we can see that Thai massage today shares much with yogic ideas common to the Tantric layer of Indian culture, post-dating the biography of Jivaka by at least 1000 years and the Ayurvedic ideas discussed in the previous chapter by at least several centuries. The practice of massage also reveals significant Chinese influence, as we will see in the latter part of this chapter.

Tantra and Hatha-Yoga

The merger of Buddhism and medicine in India is exemplified by the Tantric texts. Tantra was an extremely popular pan-Asian phenomenon that began to emerge in the sixth century and peaked in the early second millennium, crossing national and religious boundaries. Buddhism and Hinduism equally drew upon Tantric ideas, blending esoteric views of the body with a rich practice of visualization meditation, ritualized acts, and sexual imagery.

Tantra's model challenged Ayurveda and presented a radical new vision of health and the human body. According to Ayurvedic historian Dominik Wujastyk, the Tantric body is a

> magico-religious body [which] is the universe in miniature, and a conduit for mystical energies that awaken consciousness in the chakras. None of these concepts is present or prominent in the ayurvedic view of the body, which by contrast is a map for a doctor, who must know where the physical organs and processes reside in order to relieve the suffering of the sick.[1]

Possibly the single most important contribution of the Tantric movement to Thai medicine was the development of *hatha yoga*, the practice of assuming physical postures to affect change within the body. There is evidence that ideas about the subtle body and yogic practices were discussed in India as early as the sixth century B.C.E., for example, in the *Chandogya Upanishad*. However, it was not until the twelfth and thirteenth centuries C.E., that Hindu texts such as the *Goraksha-Paddhati* blended Tantric views of the body with Upanishadic philosophy, and articulated a system similar to what we know today as *hatha yoga*.[2] Today, this system traces a network of vessels (called *nadis*) which transport the various energies created by semen (*retas*), nutritive fluids (*rasa*) and breath (*prana*). *Hatha yoga* also delineates numerous powerful points on the body (called *chakras* and *marman*) and prescribes the assumption of

1 Wujastyk (2003), p. 260.
2 Feuerstein (2001), p. 400.

physical postures (Skt. *asana*) for the generation of physical and spiritual power.

A Thai Yoga

Thai massage, as practiced today by both licensed doctors and less qualified practitioners at beauty salons and spas across the country, is a form of interactive *hatha-yoga* and acupressure based loosely on these same Tantric principles. The influence of *hatha-yoga* in Thailand is evident as early as the 1830s at Wat Pho, with the production of the *ruesri dat ton* statues described in Chapter 1. The last few years have seen a resurgence of this individualized yoga practice and its integration into the TTM curriculum. However, this practice is still relatively unknown to academics, and has yet to attract any attention in the literature.

Therapeutic Thai massage, also based on *hatha-yoga*, remains enormously popular across the country. The details tend to vary from place to place; however, most massage therapy sessions include a series of *asanas* which are performed by the therapist manipulating the patient's body into *hatha-yogic* positions. The massage is conducted on a mattress on the floor, fully clothed, typically without any oils or other lubricants. While supporting limbs and using gravity to achieve results with a minimum of effort, the therapist moves the patient through a series of postures intended to energize the body, improve flexibility and strength, and to affect the deeper energies within. Chiropractic adjustments related to the traditional Thai practice of bonesetting, *dat kraduk* or *hak kraduk*, are also a feature of most massage routines.

In addition to the *asanas* and chiropractic adjustments, another important part of Thai massage is the stimulation of pressure points (*jap sen*) along the body's 72,000 vessels (*sen*).[3]

---

3   Literally, *sen* are filaments, fibers, threads, or tendons. See McFarland (1944).

Although most agree on the importance of these vessels as conduits for subtle energies throughout the body, virtually every massage school in Thailand adheres to a different *sen* system. General theoretical principles tend to be similar, but the exact location of the *sen* and the ways in which they are treated tend to be quite idiosyncratic. Competing models of massage theory have evolved around particularly influential teachers—to the extent that it is common today to speak of different "lineages" of Thai massage centered around well-known schools such as Shivagakomarpaj, Wat Pho, or charismatic individuals like Pichest Boonthume and Lek Chaiya Thiwong in Chiang Mai, as well as among their well-known Western students such as the late Harald "Asokananda" Brust.

The language used to describe the *sen* is somewhat ambiguous. In modern Thai parlance, it is common to say that *lom* moves through the *sen* and animates the body. However, this terminology can lead to very different translations in English. On the one hand, "*lom* in the *sen*" can quite literally mean "air in the vessels." The Thai Ayurvedic texts, in fact, do claim that the air element (*lom*) literally circulates through the body, and lists under the air element parts of the body:

> air which starts at the feet and rises to the head, air which starts from the head and descends to the feet, air in the abdominal cavity, air which circulates in the intestines and stomach, air which circulates throughout the body, the breath inhaled and exhaled.[4]

It seems possible to interpret this passage as stating that breath enters the body through the nose or mouth, and moves through the vessels and tendons of the body. (This interpretation is also possible in the Indian notion of *prana* traveling in the *nadis*, which also literally means "air in the vessels," or the

---

4   See Table 4.2 for citation.

Chinese notion of *qi* in the *mai*, which is translatable as "vapor in the vessels.")

This literal circulation of air in the vessels, however, is often replaced by a metaphorical interpretation based on a loosely-defined network of subtle energy. For the most part, traditional Thai therapists I worked with tended to state that there is an intangible, invisible force called *lom* which, moving through non-anatomical energetic pathways, can be manipulated through directed pressure and conscious intent on the part of the practitioner. The goal of moving or stimulating the *lom* is to offer both therapy and the maintenance of health. The *sen* are treated with thumb pressure along the channels, and with repeated pressure on certain important points located on the lines.

At Shivagakomarpaj, it is taught that there are ten main *sen* lines treated for different symptoms and diseases, and that virtually any disorder may be treated with massage. Massage will invariably be utilized as the principal treatment, or as an adjunct therapy for the hospital's patients, even when the primary complaint of the patient is not a mechanical issue. Massage, for example, is indicated for cancer, HIV-AIDS, and other chronic systemic conditions. Additionally, a full-body treatment of all ten main *sen* on a regular basis is said to promote longevity and well-being. This therapy is particularly favored among Thais of the older generations, who—along with tourists—make up the bulk of the clientele at Chiang Mai massage clinics.

The connections between the Thai *sen* and the yogic Indian *nadis*, as they are presented in popular contemporary Ayurvedic manuals, are intriguing. Although they do not always run exactly the same course, several of these *sen* share closely cognate names and similar locations. For example, *pingala nadi* (Skt.) correlates closely with *sen pingala* (Th.), both of which originate from the navel and terminate at the right nostril. *Ida nadi* (Skt.) and *sen ida* (Th.) terminate at the left. *Sushumna nadi* (Skt.)

and *sen sumana* (Th.) follow the spinal cord. See Table 5.1 for a summary of these correlations.

TABLE 5.1. COMPARISON OF TERMINAL ORIFICES FOR *SEN* AND *NADIS*

Terminal orifices	Thai *sen*	Indian *nadis*[5]
Left nostril	Ida	Ida
Right nostril	Pingala	Pingala
Left eye	Sahatsarangsi	Ghandari
Right eye	Tawari	Pusha
Left ear	Lawusang	Shankhini
Right ear	Ulanga	Payasvini
Urethra	Nantakawat	Kuhu
Anus	Kitcha	Alambusha
Right fingers and toes	Kalathari	Yashasvati
Left fingers and toes	Kalathari	Hastijihva
Mouth	Sumana	Sushumna (follows same course but terminates at crown)

5   Abridged from Frawley (1999), p. 157-161.

A Diversity of Practices

The Wat Pho tablets, while being recognized as the official basis of Thai massage theory, do not exert a standardizing influence in practice. It is apparent from even a quick survey of the student manuals of the main massage schools in Thailand today that the practice of massage is nowhere near consistent from place to place.[6] While a national curriculum exists for the education of herbalists based on authoritative texts, the massage curriculum tends to vary rather widely from school to school—particularly on theoretical matters. While efforts to standardize this therapy have been undertaken in the past few years (I present more on this in the final chapter of this book), massage is still very much a regional practice colored by a diversity of influences. In Thailand today, one finds a wide range of therapies at many hotels, spas, massage clinics, and traditional medical centers.

In many schools of therapeutic massage one can find much Chinese influence. As shown in Table 5.1 above, Shivagakomarpaj attributes much of the system of *sen* and postures to *hatha yoga*, and in many cases utilizes Sanskrit terminology and names. Despite the shared nomenclature, however, the actual pathways of the *sen* channels used at this school often bear as much similarity to Chinese acupuncture meridians as to Indian *nadis*. Though the starting and ending points stay true to the yoga *nadis*, comparing the charts in Figs. 5 and 6, we can see that the path of the Thai *sen* through the back, legs, and arms actually seem to connect pieces of Chinese meridians. The charts in Fig. 7-8 likewise show the overlaps between Thai, Indian, and Chinese point systems, indicating that Shivagakomarpaj's massage theory draws equally on both systems.

6   Manuals consulted for this comparison include the basic massage student manuals for three well-known Chiang Mai massage schools, Chaichakan (1997), Setthakorn (1997), and Thiwong (1997), as well as four published books associated with three other Chiang Mai massage schools, Chaithavuthi and Muangsiri (2005), Asokananda (1990), and Apfelbaum (2004).

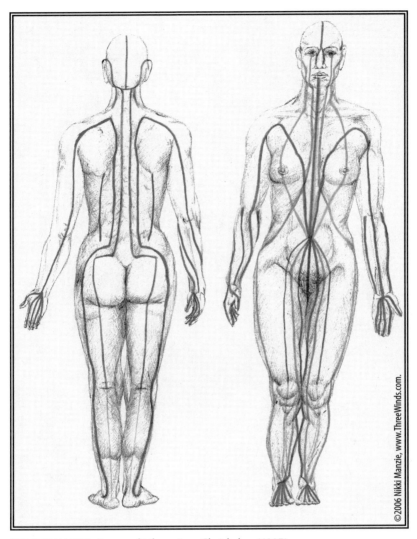

©2006 Nikki Manzie, www.ThreeWinds.com.

FIG. 5. THAI *SEN*   *Source of information: Chaichakan (1997).*

Although the Shivagakomarpaj theory of massage does not include the concepts of *yin-yang*, the Five Phases, or the relation of *sen* to organs familiar from Chinese medicine, when it comes to practice, still there are many close similarities between these two traditions. Leaving aside the postures from *hatha yoga*, *nuad boran* as it is practiced today resembles closely a number

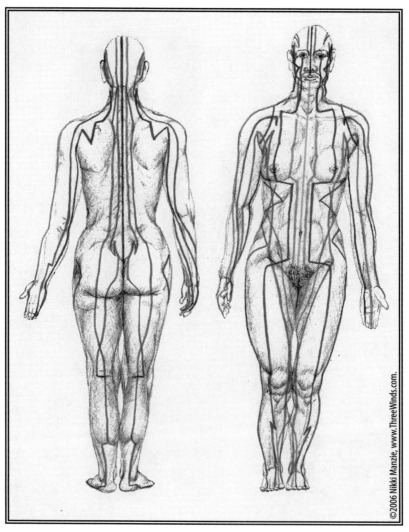

©2006 Nikki Manzie, www.ThreeWinds.com.

FIG. 6. TCM MERIDIANS

of other East Asian therapies such as *tuina* and *shiatsu*. *Nuad boran* focuses on stimulation of the *sen* in a manner similar to Chinese meridian work, and is often termed "Thai acupressure." Moreover, most modern Thai massage schools, including both Shivagakomarpaj as well as Wat Pho, freely utilize Chinese reflexology and acupressure point charts in their curriculum,

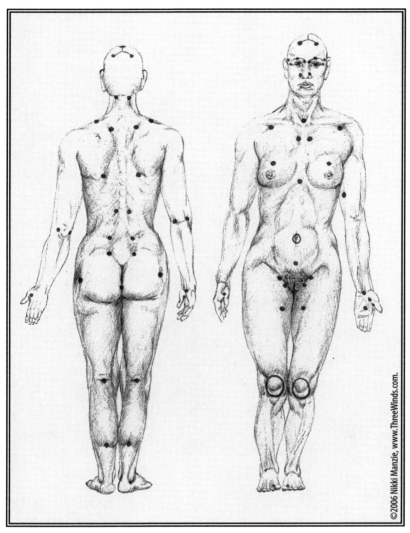

FIG. 7. COMPARATIVE CHARTS: THAI *JAP SEN* POINTS SHARED WITH INDIAN *MARMA* POINTS   *Source of information on Thai points: Chaichakan (1997).*

and even have developed "Thai foot massage" courses based on Chinese models.

Whether these correlations are the product of Chinese influence in Thailand, or whether both the Chinese and the Thai systems share common roots in a greater Asian tradition remains a matter for speculation. As there are no records of

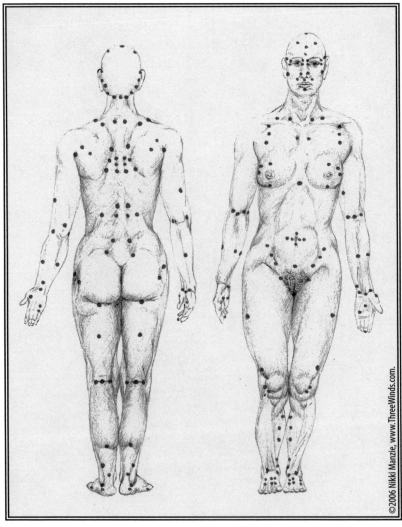

FIG. 8. COMPARATIVE CHARTS: THAI *JAP SEN* POINTS SHARED WITH CHINESE ACUPCUNTURE POINTS   *Source of information on Thai points: Chaichakan (1997).*

Thai massage therapy before the Wat Pho stone tablets, and while these remain untranslated, we simply can not know. Nonetheless, *nuad boran* can be said to be—like much of Thai medicine—a syncretic blend, combining features of more than one system.

PART III

Diversity in
Traditional Thai Medicine

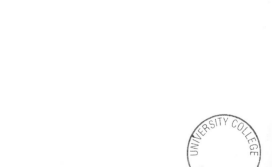

CHAPTER 6

Thai Folk Healing

The Buddhist rituals, Ayurvedic humoral/elemental philosophy, Tantric-influenced yogic postures, and Chinese acu-point therapy presented thus far are united in apparent theoretical consistency in TTM but, in actuality, represent quite different ways of thinking about the body. We have thus far been emphasizing the literate tradition and have found TTM to be an amalgam of eclectic practices. If one even just scratches the surface of the non-literate practices, Thai healing reveals a wealth of diversity unrelated to Ayurveda, yoga, or TCM. These practices are not part of the elite, learned system of the *mo boran* regulated by the Ministry of Public Health, but remain an important part of healthcare in Thailand today. In this chapter, I will discuss a small sample of the practices native to Southeast Asia, and I will widen the scope of the discussion to include Chinese influences as well.

Two Thai Systems, Revisited

The types of therapies that I call "folk healing" in this book, for lack of a better term, are among the most popular forms of healing in Thailand today, and require considerable attention in any book on Thai medicine. Although, in the Thai case, it has been common to denigrate folk practices as "rural medicine," healers dealing in magic and spiritual forces remain among the most frequently-consulted types of practitioners of medicine even among wealthy social circles in the Thai cities. The problems with the rural/urban and elite/folk divisions have been discussed in the Introduction to this book. Perhaps a better way of approaching the seemingly bifurcated fields of Thai medicine is, instead of focusing on the regional or social differences between practitioners, to differentiate between two types of medical approaches.

Paul Hinderling argues that, broadly speaking, Thai medicine embraces two etiologies.[1] On the one hand are those forms of healing that emphasize the reliance for health on the internal balance of impersonal cosmic forces, such as elements and *doshas*, and that see imbalance as the cause of disease. These practices draw from the Ayurvedic and yogic tradition, as well as on Theravada Buddhist philosophy. This approach to investigating natural phenomena is, in Thailand, also influenced by the traditional medicine of China. These types of therapies, for the most part, are the purview of physicians who are highly educated, or other members of a professional class of healers. Most modern Thais consult a panoply of specialists in this category when illness or misfortune falls, including formally-trained *mo boran*, massage therapists, traditional pharmacists, herbalists, and Chinese doctors.

On the other hand, Thai medicine also incorporates many practices which are not concerned with internal balance but with external agency and see disease as an attack from without. While the Ayurvedic or Chinese physician counsels balance and moderation, the practitioners of demonological healing arts cultivate beneficial magical powers and spirit-allies and protect the patient against attack by malevolent invisible forces such as ghosts, evil spirits, and sorcery. These healing practices center on beliefs which bear some similarity to demonological systems from many other cultures across Asia. Although we should not equate medical systems from vastly different contexts, we

1   See Hinderling (1973), p. 12, for a discussion of this idea.

should note that similar demonological ideas can be found in early China and India, as well as among many contemporary Southeast Asian groups.[2]

It is also interesting to note the similarities between demonological medicine and modern biomedicine. Although these two types of medicine may seem at first blush to belong to opposite ends of the spectrum, both share an etiology that understands disease as a result of an attack on the body by unseen entities that need to be eradicated, and the maintenance of health as a continual process of warding off such attacks. This similarity has enabled many of biomedicine's therapeutic strategies to be co-opted by folk healers, such as in the case of the injection doctors I mentioned in Chapter 3.

The Thai Spirit World

Thai folk cosmology includes many beneficial and many dangerous forces. These powers are outlined in Table 6.1, which lists forces always dangerous, forces always beneficial, and those that are ambiguous, or which can be used for either good or evil. The manipulation of these various forces is the purview of the *mo ratsadon* or *mo tjaloe* (which Heinze translates as "folk-practitioner").[3] These healers include the *mo du* (fortune teller or astrologer), *mo song* (diviner), and the *mo wicha* (controller of magical power).[4] Other ritual specialists may include monks, who are considered powerful and auspicious beings. Additionally, Thai Brahmins specialize in astrology, weddings, state ceremonies, and mediation with Hindu deities who are considered important *thewada*, or demi-gods, by many Thais.[5]

---

2   For demonology in China, see Harper (1985); for India, see Zysk (1993a); for Southeast Asia, see Heinze (1997).

3   Heinze (1977), p. 91.

4   Heinze (1977), p. 91. The word *mo* in all these instances can be translated as "doctor" or "healer."

5   Heinze (1992), p. 18.

TABLE 6.1. THE RANGE OF MYSTICAL POWERS IN THAI COSMOLOGY[6]

Dangerous	Ambiguous	Beneficial
corpses	gods	meditation
evil spirits (*phi*)	ancestors	Pali chants
excreta	guardian spirits (*khwan*)	amulets
tall trees	books on astrology	monk's implements (e.g. bowls, other sacred objects)
dark places	healing arts	
aggressive magic		

Anthropologists typically understand such practices as being un-theorized "ritual technologies." While sometimes drawing on sacred literature, symbols, and rituals, the healing arts of the practitioners dealing in these invisible forces are not typically based on learned ideas or coherent philosophies. Likewise, these are not organized professionals regulated by government agencies, but charismatic individuals with idiosyncratic styles of therapy and unique notions of disease etiology and nosology (cause and classification). Even when these practitioners are ordained monks, their healing arts usually do not rest on

6   Abridged from Terwiel (1976), p. 400. Parentheses are mine.

Buddhist texts and are often in conflict with the orthodox religious philosophy. Nevertheless, folk-healing—far from being a separate endeavor from religious practice—remains an important feature of Thai popular religion, despite the internal tension and inconsistencies this combination frequently raises.

Thai Phi

Thai folk-healing owes much to indigenous T'ai belief predating Indian influence in Southeast Asia. Indeed, similarities in ceremonies and ritual paraphernalia can be found among groups of T'ais throughout the remoter regions of Southeast Asia, some of which have never been exposed to much Indian culture.[7] One common feature of almost all T'ai groups is a strong belief in ghosts (*phi*) as a source of misfortune and disease. The Thai belief in *phi* is quite strong, even among many of the most educated and sophisticated urbanites today.[8]

In Thailand, *phi* are believed to be created through an "unfortunate death," one that is untimely or particularly sudden. Upon sudden death, the *phi* may not be aware of the passing away of the body, and may continue to live in the human realm indefinitely. Other *phi*, particularly if there was an injustice or crime involved, may refuse to be reborn, and instead choose to continue to live on earth and wreak havoc on humankind in a quest for vengeance. The most terrifying *phi* is the *phi t'ai hong*, or the *phi* of the person who has died violently, for it can be both vengeful and violent. Locations where *phi* tend to be found include graveyards, forests, ponds (especially those in which someone has drowned), and other places where misfortune or death has struck.

Often, attack by a *phi* manifests in its victim as an incurable, undiagnosable, or terminal illness. Symptoms of *phi* diseases

---

7 See Terwiel (1978a).
8 See Hinderling (1973) for information on *phi* in this section.

also include common ailments such as headache, dizziness, diarrhea, sudden loss of weight, sudden painful swelling, menstrual complications, and so forth, which do not respond to medications or other therapies.[9] It is also possible that a *phi* would possess an individual, assuming control of the victim's body and speech in order to express its grievances to the community. (This explanation could be used, for example, in cases of what Western medicine would diagnose as schizophrenia or other psychological diseases.) It is often the case when an individual has died unjustly or by the fault of another that the dead person's *phi* possesses individuals in his or her community in search of justice until the matter is redressed or the death is avenged. Normally, this type of *phi* attack is temporary, and the possessed return to normalcy after the grievances are addressed.

Dealing with the world of the *phi* is the specialty of two different groups of practitioners.[10] The *mo phi* (spirit medium) is responsible for maintaining harmony between the human world and that of the *phi*. The *mo phi* ensures that these ghosts are adequately taken care of so that they leave humans alone, and provide the *phi* with the ability to make their needs known to the community. These spirit mediums fall into several categories, including the *makhi*, whose body becomes fully possessed by a spirit while the practitioner's soul travels to the heavens. These mediums do not stay conscious during their possession, and do not remember what transpires. Other mediums maintain some control over their physical bodies, while still others are channels for the spoken words of spirits while maintaining full consciousness and control.

The *mo phi pob*, on the other hand, is a healer who assists victims of attack or possession by these dangerous spirits. These healers tame and pacify malevolent *phi* with various tools. Many use consecrated water (*nam mon*) to induce *phi* to speak, the

---

9   Hinderling (1973), p. 27.
10 See Heinze (1992), p. 19, for information in this section.

thinking being that once a *phi* expresses itself it may leave voluntarily. Others utilize a "blowing" technique common to many forms of shamanism worldwide by which *phi* are thought to be blown out of the body.[11] Other implements include magically-charged tools that symbolically capture, punish, or destroy the *phi*. Table 6.2 below lists the tools available to different types of healers to assist them to deal with the spirit world.

Not all *phi* are necessarily evil, however. While the unfortunate dead are always a source of anxiety in the Thai spiritual world, *phi* can be quite helpful if properly managed, and may

TABLE 6.2. THAI HEALERS AND THEIR THERAPEUTIC TOOLS AGAINST PHI[12]

Type of healer	Action
anyone	demand that it leave
minor exorcist	ceremony with candles and incense-sticks
monk	strengthening by prayer and meditation
mo phi (or *mo phi pob*) or occasionally *mo boran*	holy water or "blowing"
mo phi (or *mo phi pob*) only	fight if *phi* resists; use implements like magic knife, whip, helping spirits, foods such as flour

11 Hinderling (1973), p. 47, 49.
12 Abridged from Hinderling (1973), p. 34. Parentheses are mine.

be cultivated by practitioners of magic (Th. *saiyasath*) as familiars or spiritual allies. While some beneficial *phi* are of human origin, others seem to be personifications of objects in nature, and therefore lead many scholars to refer to the belief in *phi* and the practices associated with their pacification as "Thai animism." Potentially beneficial *phi* are listed in Table 6.3.

TABLE 6.3. POTENTIALLY BENEFICIAL *PHI*[13]

Phi Soo-a Wat, spirits of deceased Buddhist monks, which are now protective spirits of temples

Phi paa, jungle spirits

Phi khau, mountain spirits

Phi nang mai, female tree-spirits

Phi pluak, termite spirits

Phi muang, town-spirits

Phra Phum Chaeo Thi, the spirit of the land

Phi khru, spirits of one's teacher

The second to last *phi* in Table 6.3, the spirit of the land, or the earth-spirit, is quite popular in Thai folk religion. Most Thai homes, offices, hotels, and other buildings include an area where the earth-spirit displaced by human construction is allowed to reside (see Fig. 9). In most cases, this is a small bird-house-like construction, usually elevated on a post, which is in the shape of a well-to-do home or palace. These spirit-

13 This table is abridged from Hinderling (1973), p. 25, and Heinze (1982), p. 27-30.

houses are tended on a daily basis in a ceremony known as *wai phi* (or honoring the *phi*), whereby offerings of incense, water, fruit, rice, and other foodstuffs are given in order to placate the resident *phi*. It is believed that it is essential to keep all *phi* happy, as an unhappy ghost can cause calamity and disease in the home or financial disaster in business. The *wai phi* is a very common daily practice among Thais in all socioeconomic settings. In the villages and Bangkok suburbs alike, on college campuses and in resort hotels, the morning propitiation of the spirits can be seen. When it comes to the spirit world, it seems that prevention is the best form of medicine.

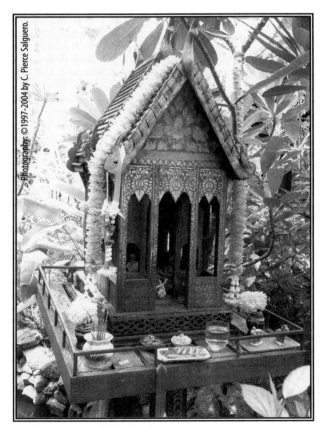

FIG. 9. A HOUSE FOR *PHI*, KOH SAMUI.

Buddhism, Popular Religion and the Jivaka Ritual

The last *phi* on the list in Table 6.3 reminds us of the discussion of the *wai khru* ceremonies from Chapter 2. In that chapter, I outlined the ceremony Thai healers use to honor the "Father Doctor" Jivaka as the founder of the lineage of Thai medicine. Other practitioners of traditional arts and crafts also celebrate and dedicate rituals to their deceased teachers. Whether the subject of the propitiatory rituals is Jivaka or another teacher (mythical or historical), the *wai khru* ceremony is a type of *wai phi* ceremony.

While the oral and written texts, statues, architecture, and rituals associated with Jivaka serve to legitimize the practice of traditional Thai medicine through identification with a figure from Buddhist scripture, the Jivaka *wai khru* ritual positions him as a powerful ally in the popular Thai cosmology and make visible the supernatural powers the healer draws from his lineage of deceased teachers. Although the Jivaka *wai khru* utilizes Buddhist imagery and language, the purpose of the ceremony—to honor a teacher with chanting, offerings, and gifts, both to keep them happy in the spirit world and to enable the practitioner to call upon their powers to assist in performing certain tasks on earth—is similar to the treatment of other *phi* in the Thai pantheon.

The *wai khru* is not merely understood symbolically. The performance of the *wai khru* is an invocation of Jivaka's *phi* as a supernatural aid in healing. Like the kick-boxer calling on his master's ghost to help him win a match, or the exorcist calling on a spirit-helper to assist in repelling a malevolent ghost, Jivaka's *wai khru* ceremony calls forth the Buddha's doctor's presence in order to guide the practitioner in the act of healing. This interpretation was asserted by my interviewees among massage practitioners at Shivagakomarpaj, who reported that they believed Jivaka was present during their sessions with patients, and transmitted healing "through" their hands. One prominent massage teacher in Chiang Mai formerly associated with the hospital expressed the meaning of the Jivaka *wai khru* thus: "Through this prayer, we request [Jivaka's] help, that through our hands, [he] will bring wholeness and health to the body of our client."[14]

The paradoxical use of Jivaka in this ritual is a particularly striking example in which we can see the categories employed by scholars—such as elite/folk, Buddhist/animist, Indic/indigenous, or even the distinction between medicine and religion—do not make much sense as analytical categories in discussing contemporary Thai healing practice.[15] The use of Jivaka by traditional healers resists description in these simple binary terms, leading the observer to conclude that we must analyze the multivalency of symbols in order to understand the complex ways in which Jivaka speaks to the people who invoke him in their daily lives.

Thai Yan, Tattoos, and Amulets

Thai yan, or magical charms, are elaborate mystical symbols, geometric designs reminiscent of Tantric yantras and mandalas, or of Chinese magical seals.[16] Yan can be found in places where they can bestow protection on their owners or wearers, such as in doorways, on dashboards, and around one's neck. Thai yan consist of syllables from the Khmer alphabet, numerology, images of Buddhas, folk-deities and heroes, and powerful symbolic animals such as lions, tigers, and turtles. These elements are arranged in geometrical patterns—predominantly squares,

14 From translation of *wai khru* ceremony by Chonggkol Setthakorn, Chaichakan (1997), frontispiece.
15 See Terwiel (1976) for an alternate model for analysis of Thai popular Buddhism that does not rely on these types of cateories.
16 One of the best sources on Thai amulets is Tambiah (1984). See Strickmann (2002) for examples of medical uses of Chinese talismans and seals.

circles, and triangles—with esoteric meanings attached to each configuration (see Fig. 10).

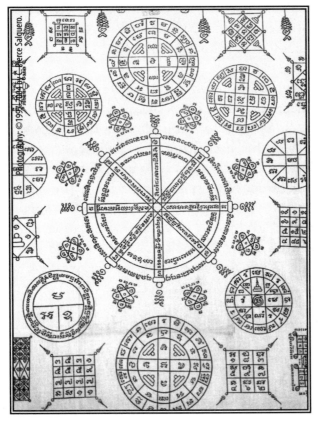

FIG. 10. *YAN* DEPICTING KHMER ALPHABET AND GEOMETRIC SYMBOLS.

The Khmer script used in *yan* is held by Thais to be particularly sacred or magically powerful. However, among my friends who were interested in *yan* in Chiang Mai, there were none who could identify more than a few syllables of the Khmer writings. Nevertheless, they were in general agreement that the script was powerful in and of itself. Though most could not interpret specific elements of the *yan*, the overall meaning of an individual charm seemed to be well known. This observation suggests that these designs are less important for their actual

80

content than for their more general acquired meaning and their association with mystical symbolism. This is consistent with many practices in Esoteric Buddhism and other Tantric traditions, in which it is precisely the exoticism and mysteriousness inherent in the practices that give them their power. As one friend recently explained it, "the less you know about how it works, the more powerful the *yan*."[17]

The art of tattooing is another popular use for these protective symbols. This practice is probably related to a greater tradition of body art prevalent across Southeast Asia, Southern China, Polynesia, and as far away as New Zealand among the Maori. Throughout this large region, tattoos serve as markers of manhood, and the procurement of a tattoo is considered a rite of passage for young men. Ancient Chinese sources speak of men from *Yue* (usually understood to refer to Southeast Asia) tattooing their faces, so there is a high degree of likelihood that tattooing as a practice is quite old in this region. There is evidence that tattoos enjoyed a high level of popularity in Thailand even in recent history. Phya Rajadhon wrote that in the early 1900s, he remembered "most Thai men were tattooed, many from waist to knees."[18] Protective tattoos are still popular among Thai men, particularly those involved in high-risk employment such as policemen and soldiers, and remain a particularly potent symbol of masculinity.

Another important type of charm is the amulet, or *khawng-khlang*. While natural objects such as precious stones, trees that were struck by lightning, or plants that look like Buddhas have inherent magical powers, artificial objects can also be imbued with such powers as well.[19] The most powerful amulets are made by mixing in a base of resin the ashes or relics of cremated masters. Images of Buddhas, often copies of existing statues

---

17 Wit Sukhsamran, personal communication.
18 Rajadhon (1964), p. 186.
19 Chirapravati (1997), p. 68. See Chapter 6 as well as Rajadhon (1964) for information in this paragraph.

with reputations for being auspicious, are then stamped into the resin, and hung around the neck. Cremation of books is common when sacred Buddhist texts have outlived their usefulness, and these ashes can also be mixed into an amulet's ingredients. Even if these special ashes are not used in their fabrication artificial amulets can be powerful. They may be made of metal, plastic, or any material, and can be activated through the ceremony of *pluk sek* to "charge them" with beneficial protective magical power.[20]

The use of this type of magic in Thailand is usually associated with certain taboos. Amulets, tattoos, and other *yan* typically come with restrictions the bearer must respect against certain foods such as beef, pork, certain vegetables, or even foods of a particular texture. It is common practice among folk-healers to not accept fees for healing services, to avoid alcohol, or to avoid meat.[21] In most cases, taboos are equivalent to power, and the more magic power one wields, the more restrictive the taboos one follows. The most powerful kind of taboos are those that have a foundation in Buddhism. Because monks must follow the 227 rules of the monastic code, they are seen as being among the most powerful beings (monks rank above even the *thewada*, or demi-gods, in the cosmic hierarchy).[22] Forest monks, who are generally thought to practice much more diligently than their city counterparts, are considered to be even more auspicious for they often take on additional ascetic austerities (such as only eating once a day) which are optional to the monkhood and are rarely followed in the city. If one can not live the monastic life—and most folk-healers do not—one may still follow the principles of *sila* (morality). *Sila* is exemplified by observing the five Buddhist precepts: refraining from killing, stealing, dishonesty, sexual misconduct, and intoxicants.

---

20 Rajadhon (1964), p. 178.
21 Suwanlert (1976), p. 69.
22 Tannenbaum (1993), p. 72.

Sometimes individual minor points of monastic discipline are extracted from the monastic code to serve as taboos as well, such as the restriction against walking under a clothesline. In general, the idea seems to be that magical powers can only be utilized successfully by one who exhibits self-control through avoidance of certain activities, and that continuous attention to self-control enhances magical powers.[23]

Gatha

Another Thai healing practice that has roots in the larger Indic religious milieu, but which is often classified as folk healing, is the chanting of *gatha*. *Gatha* are related to *mantra* and *dharani*, practices of chanting sacred syllables common to Mahayana and Tantric Buddhism as well as to Hindu tradition.[24] *Gatha* in Thailand are spells used to harness sacred and magical powers. *Gatha* typically accompany amulets and yan, and, when chanted, are thought to enhance the protection offered by such charms. *Gatha* can also be chanted by healers and shamans of any kind, including exorcists, tattooists, as well as herbalists and massage doctors to enhance the healing powers of their therapies.

In principle, any phrase with sacred meaning or any section of Buddhist scripture may be used as a *gatha*, however, in practice there are specific *gatha* for specific purposes, such as the chant to invoke and regulate the four elements reproduced below in Table 6.4. Each phrase in the *gatha* below repeats the words *Namo Buddhaya*, or "Homage to the Buddha." The syllables *na*, *ma*, *ba*, and *da*, each representing one of the four elements, are then rearranged in order to prioritize the element being called upon.

---

23 For a more theoretical discussion about the relationship between taboos and magical power discussed in this section, see Tannenbaum (1993).
24 See discussion of the power of the sacred word in Thailand in Hinderling (1973), p. 38-42.

TABLE 6.4. *GATHA* FOR THE FOUR ELEMENTS[25]	
Water: NAMO BUDDHAAYA NA MA BA DA NAMO BUDDHAAYA	**Fire:** NAMO BUDDHAAYA BA DA NA MA NAMO BUDDHAAYA
Earth: NAMO BUDDHAAYA MA BA DA NA NAMO BUDDHAAYA	**Wind:** NAMO BUDDHAAYA DA NA MA BA NAMO BUDDHAAYA

This *gatha* is quite simple, and the meaning is quite clear. More complex *gatha* may include lengthy repetitions of seemingly nonsensical syllables, and again, the performer of the chant is not required (or encouraged) to understand the meaning for it to be efficacious. An example of the application of this type of *gatha* could be in the preparation of herbal medicines for the regulation of one of the elements that had fallen out of balance. The herbalist may chant the appropriate *gatha* while preparing the medicine, and may even wrap the medicine within a paper depicting a *yan* in order imbue it with even more powers.

The Tham Khwan *Ceremony*

Another very common folk-healing custom with links to T'ai indigenous practice is the *tham khwan*, or "calling of the soul." It is not known how old this practice is, but as different variations on this ritual can be found throughout East and Southeast Asia—including among virtually all groups of T'ai people, as well as many other ethnic groups in the area—it is probably of quite ancient origin. In the Thai *tham khwan* ceremony, the *khwan*, the soul or guardian spirit of an individual,

25 Source: Wit Sukhsamran, personal communication.

is believed to have been lost, leading to disease and mental stress. The soul is called back home by a *mo khwan* (or soul doctor), or by an elder in the family or village.

According to Ruth-Inge Heinze, the Thais have many different terms for a wide variety of concepts which might be translatable as "soul" in English (see Table 7.1).[26] Note that this list includes both cognate words drawn from Indian and Chinese ideas. Heinze and other scholars specifically draw linguistic connections between the Thai *khwan* and the Chinese *hun* (made up of the characters for demon and cloud), which are presumed to be related concepts.[27] The *hun* is a

TABLE 7.1. THAI "SOULS"

Thai word	English translation	Cognate
khwan	essence	Chinese *hun*
vinyan	perception, consciousness	Pali *viññana*
citta	intuition, mind	Pali *citta*
ming	good fortune, prosperity	Chinese *ming*
citaphud	shadow, reflection	?
upanidsaj	ingrained character	Pali *nidsanj*
phron likhid	individual karma	?

26 The English word "soul" is used here rather loosely, noting Theravada Buddhist philosophy's rejection of an eternal *atta* (Skt. *atman*), or a soul in the Judeo-Christian sense of the word.
27 Heinze (1977), p. 93 and Rajadhon (1962), p. 120.

Chinese word for the soul of the individual which becomes detached from the body upon death and returns as a ghost. In Thailand, the *khwan* is seen as a "guardian spirit," or as the "essence of life," a personification of the individual's vitality and strength.[28]

Not only humans but trees, animals, houses, and entire cities are thought to have *khwan*.[29] These khwan can furthermore be male or female: for example, the spirit of a tree which is useful for building is typically female, while trees that are not utilized in this way (such as banyan) are typically male.[30] The number of khwan in the human body is usually thirty-two, each residing in a different part of the body drawn from the list of body parts given in the Earth and Water sections of Table 4.2.[31] The wellbeing of each of these *khwan* can have a direct relationship to the overall health of the individual.

In Thai belief, the *chai*, or the *khwan* of the heart, is the most important one, and the one which receives most attention in healing rituals. It is commonly believed that this *khwan* can become dislodged from the body due to trauma either physical or psychological, and can become lost, unable to return to its rightful place. Children seem to be especially susceptible to this type of occurrence. For example, a child who receives a fright or a shock of some kind may be considered to have lost his or her *khwan*. If it is not recovered, the loss of a *khwan* is said to lead to dizziness, fatigue, fevers and other symptoms, which eventually develop into madness and even death.[32]

---

28 Heinze (1982), p. 17.

29 Information in this section is drawn from Rajadhon (1962) and Heinze (1977, 1982).

30 Rajadhon (1962), p. 120.

31 Heinze (1977), p. 92 note 11. As mentioned above, these parts of the body appear in both Indian and Thai tradition, so it is not particularly surprising to see them again here in this context.

32 Although we can describe specific symptoms with Western terminology, there is no adequate translation for the loss of the *khwan*. This illness, known to anthropologists as "fright," is an example of a culture-bound syndrome, or a culturally-specific disease without a Western medical counterpart.

In the ceremony of the *tham khwan*, the lost soul is called to reunite with its body. In the Thai ritual, this includes chanting and calling after the soul, offering it sweets to tempt it to return, and the binding of the right wrist (or both wrists) with consecrated thread in order to metaphorically tie the *khwan* to the body. The officiator is to repeat the phrase "Oh! *Khwan*, abide with the body!" or some variation on this exhortation.[33] In addition to occasions of healing, this ceremony is also performed as a rite of passage at certain times in life to preemptively prevent the loss of the *khwan*. These events include the first haircut of a baby, before ordination as a Buddhist monk, at marriage, returning home after a long absence or recovery from a long illness, or after a life crisis such as a change in status or residence.[34] In this type of ritual, the string is often tied to the left wrist as opposed to the right.

The Thai tham *khwan* ceremony demonstrates marked similarity with healing rites of many peoples in Southeast Asia, including the Shan, the Cambodians, the Lao, and the Hmong.[35] It is possible that all of these similarities are signs of more recent borrowing, but it appears that this is a very ancient pan-Asian rite. The earliest description of a calling of the soul ceremony I know of is found in the ancient literature of the Chinese. The Chinese ceremony apparently was utilized after the death of an individual, to attempt to call the soul back into the body and revive the corpse, and is in broad outline quite similar to the Southeast Asian rite. In the *Zhao Hun*, composed between 277 and 263 B.C.E., one finds the following description:

> A soul-summoner must take a suit of court robes formerly worn by the deceased,... and in this manner, setting a

33 Rajadhon (1962), p. 150.
34 Heinze (1977), p. 94.
35 See Fadiman (1998) for a very readable instance of this rite among Hmong refugees in America.

ladder against the east end of the front eaves of the house, is to mount up on the ridge of the roof, and there, facing northwards and stretching out the clothing, to call three times in a loud voice, "Ho, Such a One! Come back!" Then he is to hand the clothing down... And this other one, going into the room where the deceased lies, is to lay the clothing down upon the corpse.[36]

Though different in many details, this ceremony bears important similarities with the Thai *tham khwan*, such as the exhortation to the soul, the use of cloth as a vehicle for capturing the soul, and the laying of this cloth on the body to return the soul to its rightful owner. The summoning of the soul in the above-mentioned passage seems to have been a Southern Chinese tradition, and may share the same roots as the *tham khwan* in a larger Southeast Asian cultural practice.

Thai-Chinese Ghost Pacification Rituals

The importance of Chinese religious and social institutions in contemporary Thailand has already been discussed to some extent in Chapter 3. Chinese influences and practices are emphasized during the important Chinese festivals which punctuate the religious calendar. One widely celebrated holiday for Thai-Chinese temples is the Hungry Ghost Festival.[37] Temples stagger the celebration of this event throughout the seventh month so that the public can attend all of the local ceremonies. The purpose of this ritual is to offer food and paper objects to the deceased who have no descendents or who have been neglected, and are therefore suffering in the other world. These ceremonies are often large public performances of traditional Chinese rituals, and are attended by

36 Hawkes (1985), p. 219.
37 Hill (1992), p. 323. See this article for information in this paragraph.

Chinese and Thais alike, although Thais are seldom allowed to participate.

Another very visible example of the complex interplay between Chinese and Thai communities is the ritual of the refinement of restless ghosts.[38] This ceremony reflects the syncretic nature of Thai folk practice in its combination of Chinese rituals and Confucian social hierarchies, with Theravada Buddhist institutions and indigenous cosmology. The ceremony also highlights the symbiotic relationship between Chinese and Thai populations.

The cooperation between Chinese and Thais for the performance of this ritual stems from the coincidence of both cultures' belief in ghosts. There are important differences in the Thai and Chinese conceptions of ghosts.[39] As we have explored earlier in this chapter, Thais believe that *phi* are caused by violent or untimely death. In traditional Chinese understanding, ghosts are those individuals who died without leaving progeny to carry out the required Confucian ancestral rituals. Despite the practical and philosophical differences, however, the two cultures meet in the need to propitiate the ghosts of the unfortunate dead, and to escort them to their final resting place in order to protect humans from their dangerous influence.

To the Thai, the unfortunate dead are much more of a source of terror than to the Chinese, who are motivated mainly by sentiments of pity and compassion. Their fear causes the Thai to shun the unfortunate dead for fear of contamination.[40] Chinese benevolent associations, on the other hand, provide the service of burying the abandoned dead of the Thai in Chinese cemeteries. Chinese associations apparently perform this service in staggering numbers: in the space of thirteen years, just one

38 See Formoso (1996) for information presented in this section.
39 Formoso (1996), p. 220.
40 Formoso (1996), p. 221.

charitable foundation in Thailand buried the bodies of approximately 30,000 people, over half of which were children.[41]

Every five to fifteen years, a Chinese association will perform the ceremony of refinement for the benefit of the local community, during which they exhume the temporarily buried dead from their cemeteries, and perform a mass funeral and cremation, replete with rituals intended to pacify the ghosts so that they will no longer be a threat to humans. On the second day of the ceremony, effigies of the buffalo- and horse-headed assistants to the Ruler of the Underworld escort these ghosts to hell, where they are reintegrated into the cycle of *samsara* (transmigration or rebirth).[42]

This ritual is at once personal and political. The ceremony purports to improve the fate of individual ghosts, as well as to purify both the human and the unseen world. The ritual refinement of ghosts is understood to expel all dangerous ghosts from the country, and is therefore also viewed by the Thais as an essential public health service performed by the Chinese community for the wellbeing of the Thai nation. Thus, on the one hand, the public ritual of refining the ghosts serves to demonstrate the Chinese community's integration into Thai society, and their pivotal role in promoting public and national wellbeing.[43] On the other hand, however, the rituals performed as part of the ceremony are visibly Chinese in origin and form, and serve to differentiate the Chinese community from the Thai.[44] The festival is of immense importance to the Chinese community, and is therefore a rallying point for ethnic and cultural pride.

---

41 Formoso (1996), p. 221.
42 Formoso (1996), p. 228-9.
43 Formoso (1996), p. 231.
44 Formoso (1996), p. 218.

CHAPTER 7

Thai Medical Orthodoxy

Standardization and Regulation

Despite these eclectic influences described in the previous chapters, the primary materials used in the education of traditional physicians in Thailand today do not on the whole reflect Chinese, Khmer, or T'ai beliefs, but rather emphasize a system modeled on Ayurveda and *hatha-yoga*. Most of the folk practices that contributed to the formation of Thai medical culture over the centuries and make up some of its most diverse practices today are missing from the canon of tablets and texts—even though these form an important part of the actual practice both historically and in contemporary Thailand. As the tradition of TTM has become increasingly centralized and regulated, these non-standard practices have been increasingly marginalized and relegated to inferior status. I believe this process can be understood as an attempt to establish an orthodoxy (a unified theoretical basis) and an orthopraxy (a unified basis of practice) for Thai medicine based on authoritative texts at the expense of diverse non-literate traditions.

Ayurveda and *hatha-yoga* undoubtedly had been introduced to Siam long before the Bangkok period. However, judging from what sources are extant, these practices were probably not hegemonic until their revival in the Bangkok period. There is no sign of a medical orthodoxy in the Ayutthayan period. We have already noted that the medicine practiced at Ayutthaya seems to have included a variety of influences, and that a number of experts were in the employ of the king. These included Siamese, Chinese, Mon, and Western physicians. Nevertheless, by the time of the renovation of Wat Pho in the 1830s, an increased emphasis was placed on the role of Ayurvedic theory and yogic practice.

The new medical orthodoxy that emerged identified Thai medicine explicitly with Ayurveda, yoga, and Theravada Buddhism. Sometimes this was achieved by adapting texts from the Ayurvedic tradition, but, at least in several instances, this involved placing a Buddhist, yogic, or Ayurvedic veneer on pre-existing texts. For example, the *ruesri dat ton* statues discussed in Chapter 1 incorporated much Hindu iconography. Matted locks, ascetic clothing, and yogic postures belonging to a Hindu milieu, however, were brought into a Theravada Buddhist context by the manuscript that accompanied the statues. The manuscript begins with the invocation: "Saluting with both hands, we bow down before the Triple Gem which dispels all kinds of misery," an opening line that immediately associates the statues with a foundational idea of Theravada philosophy.[1]

Another example of this process of legitimization is the *Khamphi prathom chinda* (*Thai Book of Genesis*), a text in the Thai medical canon translated in its entirety in 1989 by Mulholland. Based on her translation, Mulholland concludes that "at least as far as this text is concerned, I can no longer assert that Thai traditional medicine is based primarily on the philosophy of Ayurveda."[2] She writes that the text presents "a novel system with no relationship whatsoever to Ayurvedic theory," which she feels preserves indigenous T'ai beliefs.[3] The primary concern of the text is with the *sang*, or astrological congenital diseases and weaknesses which afflict children. According to this theory, children will be susceptible to certain categories of diseases

---

1 Quoted in Griswold (1965), p. 321.
2 Mulholland (1988), p. 175.
3 Mulholland (1988), p. 179.

and will benefit from certain herbal therapies depending on their day of birth.

The *Thai Book of Genesis* is a striking example of the process by which a non-Ayurvedic text could acquire legitimacy by association with Ayurvedic ideas. Despite its decidedly non-Indian content, the *Thai Book of Genesis* was modified to fit an Ayurvedic and Buddhist mold. Being a pediatric text, it has been attributed to Jivaka. It also has throughout been overlaid with orthodox medical language. For example, the first section of the treatise contains a description of human origin, the process of conception, the labors of childbirth, and the various diseases of women and children, which is completely at odds with Buddhist mythology. Nonetheless, these passages are preceded with the "Homage to the Buddha" (already quoted above in the context of the *wai khru* ceremony), and with the following benediction:

> *namassitva ca devindam devarajasakkam iva jivakakoma-rabhaccam lokanatham tathagatham pathamacintaragan-tham bhasissam chandasomukham samkhepen kittayitam pubbe lokanam nathatthanti:* "I have paid homage to the Lord Buddha, the refuge of all the world, and then I made special obeisance to the honoured doctor Jivaka Komarabhacca whose greatness may be compared to that of the illustrious Lord Indra, the greatest of all the kings of the gods. Here is the special text on medicine on which the *Khamphee shanthasaat* is based. It was composed by master Komarabhacca long ago. In brief so that it may help all people it is set out below."[4]

Other accretions—such as certain recipes and passages mentioning the *doshas* and the four elements—have injected Ayurvedic theories into the text. Of these, Mulholland has

---

4   Mulholland (1987), p. 15.

written that they "do not sit well," and seem to have been "superimposed" either before or after sections of a text that could stand alone without any such insertions.[5] Although the dates of these interpolations are not known, it is clear that at some point an effort was made to bring a clearly non-Ayurvedic text in line with a medical tradition that valued conformity with Ayurvedic philosophy and Theravada Buddhist mythology. That a text with presumably indigenous origins would have been altered in this way indicates that the pressures to conform were stronger than the Siamese preoccupation with preserving the knowledge of their ancestors in unadulterated form.[6]

The identification of Siamese medicine with Indian models was prioritized to the extent that when Siamese medicine was codified at Wat Pho, Ayurveda and *hatha-yoga* were represented as the core of Thai medicine. At the "university in stone," it was not the practices of the T'ai, nor the Chinese, which were engraved and preserved for posterity: it was the practices with Indian pedigree.

Why did Indian medicine emerge to a position of prominence at this time? Here, I present a plausible theory: whether or not it was a conscious decision, Ayurveda seems to have fit well with the goals of the empire. The Chakri court, having faced the monumental task of rebuilding not only a kingdom but also an entire society that had been devastated by Burmese attack, and having successfully averted the threat of European colonial ambition, in the nineteenth century enjoyed one of the greatest periods of expansion. Bangkok extended its power throughout the Lanna, Lao, Khmer, and southern peninsular regions. The court considered the revival and strengthening of Siamese institutions to be central to its efforts to legitimize this revitalized and expansionist kingdom.

---

5 Mulholland (1988), p. 175.
6 Mulholland (1987), p. 12.

The Chakri kings, with some Chinese blood and Western education, seem not to have escaped being influenced in their reconstruction efforts by their contact with these other cultures: European models of universities served as the basis for the reconstructed Wat Pho, and many of the artifacts housed within demonstrate Chinese stylistic characteristics.[7] Nevertheless, the reconstruction project was fueled by a growing sense of Siamese cultural identity. The renaissance, begun with Rama I's rebuilding of the capital on the Ayutthayan model, continued with the reconstruction of Wat Pho in an attempt to showcase Siamese culture as an ancient and legitimate heritage worthy of being enshrined and displayed to the world.[8]

A revival of traditional medicine would have been part of this effort, as the standardization of medicine and a consistent medical philosophy were necessities if Thai medicine was to be upheld as a viable and equally legitimate alternative to both Western and Chinese medicine (both of which apparently had enjoyed more royal patronage at Ayutthaya if we believe de la Loubère). Emphasizing the Ayurvedic tradition would have been a logical choice for those who wished to advance a rational traditional model of medicine. Ayurveda would have been an attractive alternative in contrast to indigenous T'ai herbalism, which apparently offered little or no overarching medical theory and was a secretive tradition based on privately-held recipes, or on Chinese medicine, which was associated with a rival power. Ayurveda was empirical, extensive, ancient, and had the additional benefit of its association with Buddhism and Brahmanic state rituals. Ayurveda also had the attraction of being associated with a learned body of texts.

The court efforts to centralize and control medical practice by relying on texts for authority rather than on folk and oral tradition mirrored the process by which the court sought to

---

7   See Matics (1978) for a detailed catalogue of the objects at Wat Pho.
8   See Matics (1977) and (1978) for complete accounts of the renovations of Wat Pho.

impose a coherent structure and a textual justification for other aspects of Siamese culture during this period. The Chakri dynasty, for example, also attempted to purge heterodox folk beliefs and practices among Buddhist monastics in favor of more rational and philosophical approaches. These efforts were particularly carried out by Rama IV (r. 1851-68), who had been a monk for almost three decades before his coronation, and who attempted to replace Thai cosmology and other supernatural beliefs with a Western-influenced ethical and philosophical emphasis.[9]

Just as local non-Buddhist religious influences were challenged by a new national religious orthodoxy, a medical orthodoxy began to have a similar effect on Thailand's diverse local healing traditions. With the codification of traditional medicine at Wat Pho and the subsequent publication of authoritative medical texts upon which were based the national medical curriculum, the government began to regulate traditional medicine at the national level, and to encourage standardization. Those who would place the *mo boran* on par with their Western scientific counterparts had to dissociate Thai medicine from its so-called "superstitious" elements, and to rely increasingly on textual authority. This included the practices of all of the folk healers discussed in the previous chapters, and anyone else who was not a formally-trained *mo boran*.

Diversity in Thai Medicine Today

As we have seen, Thai herbal texts were codified in the early part of the twentieth century. The prioritization of Ayurvedic medicine crystallized in these texts has had lasting effect on the history of Thai medicine. The recent strengthening of training requirements and legislation criminalizing the practice of medicine by unlicensed massage practitioners in the 1990s has

---

9   Heinze (1992), p. 17.

called attention to the fact that this process of defining and legitimizing Thai medicine is still ongoing even today.

While Buddhist meditation and morality have been incorporated into the TTM orthodoxy, the prevalence of heterodox practices based on indigenous or other forms of folk healing has continued to be a mild embarrassment to the medical establishment and other elites who wish to promote the authoritative system of medicine formally enshrined at Wat Pho. No doubt, certain bureaus of the government recognize and value local traditions, but this view is not shared by those most aggressively promoting TTM. The Ministry of Tourism, for example, does not include exorcism or magic tattoos in its vision of Thailand as the "Medical Hub of Asia," the "Spa Capital," or the "Wellness Capital of Asia"—all phrases that can be seen ubiquitously throughout its current online promotional literature. The publications on TTM promulgated by the Ministry of Education and other government offices consulted in the course of writing this book do not mention with approval this kind of folk practice either.

Nevertheless, these practices have far from disappeared. On the contrary, while the centralized orthodox tradition was codified and regulated by the Wat Pho temple and by the relevant government offices, alternative forms of healing—such as those described in the previous chapters—continued to thrive among rich and poor in urban and rural areas alike—and in certain areas even gained ground.[10] Diverse "folk" healers today include among their ranks not only wandering mendicants and poor villagers, but also businessmen, policemen, and government officials.[11]

Despite official marginalization, in everyday terms, these folk practitioners are as representative of Thai medicine as the Ayurvedic *mo boran* or any other segment of Thai healers.

10 The Thai craze for amulets, for example, is believed to be a nineteenth- and twentieth-century phenomenon. See Chirapravati (1997), p. 66.
11 See Heinze (1997) for biographies of several high-ranking Thais who are spirit mediums.

Studies conducted by scholars in the 1970s revealed that folk medicine represented the most popular approach to medicine in Thailand.[12] Many patients consult both traditional and magical healers (and also Western-trained biomedical doctors, although these were considered by many less-affluent Thais only as a last resort[13]), and to see each as separate strata of healers serving quite separate purposes. Studies also reported that Thais use orthodox traditional medicine for physical ailments, while indigenous folk traditions for what Western biomedicine would label psychological and spiritual needs.[14]

During the 1990s and early 2000s, I have found not only that orthodox and folk medicine exist side by side, but also that they are frequently integrated within the personal healing practices of individuals on both sides of the supposed divide. In my experience, there is no clear separation between elite and folk or between literate and oral tradition in contemporary practice, but rather shades of gray where different types of knowledge and practices blend seamlessly. Among my teachers and friends in Chiang Mai's licensed medical institutions, there were none who did not participate to some extent or another in folk practices. The Thai herbalists with whom I worked—even formally-trained *mo boran* in practice of Ayurvedic forms of medicine—utilized indigenous plants, which are found only locally, and indigenous T'ai diagnostic criteria such as astrology and *sang* rather than Ayurvedic etiologies or Chinese diagnostics when prescribing herbal remedies. A study on an herbal text, the *Phrakhampi Krasai*, found much overlap between the Thai classification of diseases found in this canonical medical text and the T'ai indigenous spirit world, indicating that this integration extends even into the canonical TTM literature.[15]

12 See Hinderling (1973). I am unaware of any more recent surveys, and what changes have taken place since that time are yet to be determined.
13 Boesch (1972), p. 33.
14 Heinze (1977), p. 100.
15 Bamber (1987). This text is included in the list of canonical texts in Appendix A.

Among the massage therapists at the Shivagakomarpaj Hospital I met an astrologer, a palm-reader, and many who wore protective amulets while they worked. They invariably practiced the *wai khru* and the *wai phi* ceremonies, honoring both their Indian lineage and their indigenous spirit companions. This syncretism also worked the other way: *mo ratsadon* (folk healers) in Chiang Mai who were renowned for their abilities to communicate with spirits, to perform exorcisms, or to command magical powers, also practiced Ayurvedic herbal medicine or *hatha-yogic* massage as sidelines—some even earning considerable income and fame teaching Western tourists these techniques.

In my own field study, I have found that medicine in Thailand today is pluralistic, and Thais are still "conditioned to avoid total reliance on any single therapeutic approach."[16] In other words, the medical marketplace is still alive and well. However, I have also found that, due to pressures to regulate and standardize traditional medicine, many practitioners of non-orthodox Thai medicine are operating without legal status. Many practitioners have learned hereditary forms of healing which have been handed down orally for generations through family lineage. Due to recent strengthening of licensure requirements, these individuals are now ostensibly breaking the law when they practice their traditional arts. While the Thai government has not always strictly enforced the laws already on the books, in cities with many tourists, such as Chiang Mai, unlicensed healers are now beginning to be required to close or pay bribes to government officials to stay operational. This requirement puts financial strain on unlicensed traditional practitioners.

The struggle for orthodoxy can also be seen playing itself out in the contentious rivalries between Bangkok schools of medicine and provincial establishments outside the capital, such as Shivagakomarpaj. While the Wat Pho medical school enjoys the prestige of being affiliated with the temple that

---

16 Golomb (1985), p. 146.

houses the famous artifacts, it has sought to parlay this status into domination of the national curriculum for *mo boran*. The Shivagakomarpaj school has for decades taught a unique form of massage, and has promoted Northern Thai regional medical knowledge as a valuable tradition. However, in the past few years, even this well-established, government-licensed school has come under pressure from authorities in Bangkok for deviation from standard curricula.[17]

Since 2001, the Ministry of Public Health has forwarded an agenda at the national level of increasing standardization and bureaucratization of the practice of massage by bringing it under the purview of the existing TTM curriculum.[18] At the time of this writing, the shape of this curriculum is still to be determined, and the authoritative schools have been wrangling over these details for the past few years. No doubt, Bangkok schools such as Wat Pho will play a central role in this debate, and the final result will most likely continue the trend toward identification with Ayurveda begun in the nineteenth century.

On the one hand, the regulation has thus far had a marked effect on the legitimacy and prestige of Thai medicine both at home and abroad, and is in part responsible for the recent success the massage schools have had in attracting international students. The fact that traditional medicine is officially defined as an equally valid system alongside Western biomedicine, and the fact that the training and practice of traditional doctors have reached this degree of regulation at the national level, demonstrate the success of the centralization process. On the other hand, this process will undoubtedly continue to threaten the viability of the colorful folk traditions that make up an inseparable part of Thailand's medical heritage.

---

17 Information in the last two paragraphs is from personal communication with Wasan Chaichakan, Director of the Shivagakomarpaj Traditional Medicine Hospital, and son of the late founder, Ajahn Sintorn Chaichakan.
18 Chokevivat (2005), p. 4.

Directions for Future Research

Most records of Siamese medicine were lost in the defeat of Ayutthaya by Burma, and traditional medicine was resurrected as an integral part of a cultural renewal in the early nineteenth century. At this time, the Wat Pho temple was established with the intent to catalogue, celebrate, and preserve traditional arts in stone in the face of future external threat. Traditional medicine was included in this program as an object of national pride, a fact which need not surprise us at a time when many features of Siamese culture were being held up as both ancient and legitimate alternatives to foreign culture and science. It was at this time that medicine also began to be codified in written texts and to be regulated by the state. The result of this official support has been that, in the last two centuries, Thai medicine became an increasingly intellectual, literate endeavor with increasing standardization.

However, despite this push toward orthodoxy, Thai medicine has never been completely homogeneous in theory or practice, and it certainly is not so today. Though it is convenient to refer to aspects of traditional Thai medicine as "Thai Ayurveda" or "Thai yoga," as we have seen, Thai medicine is also characterized by its Khmer, Chinese, and indigenous T'ai features. While the identification of Thai medicine with Ayurveda and *hatha-yoga* has marginalized unlicensed practitioners and relegated them to the status of "folk healers," their diverse practices remain today a very popular and important form of healing in Thailand.

Despite current popularity, as discussed in the final chapter, the Thai government's continual push toward standardization and regulation of traditional medicine has begun to seriously threaten the extinction of folk practices found in non-elite and non-literate circles. This, however, is not the biggest threat to their existence. In my experience, the younger generations, influenced by Western culture, globalization, TV, and the internet, are for the most part not interested in learning these traditional hereditary arts. As the elder practitioners pass away, their knowledge and stories are being permanently lost, particularly in rapidly modernizing cities like Chiang Mai. Before these traditions all but disappear, there is an immediate need for academic investigation of Thai folk culture in all of its diversity. Its colorful forms of healing remain largely unknown outside of Thailand, and specifically represent a very fruitful field for further study. Very little serious work has been done in the past decades, and most of the studies on Thai folk medicine cited in this book are quite outdated.

Folk medicine notwithstanding, even the orthodox Thai medical system remains largely unstudied by the Western academic community. At the end of this book, the reader will find an extensive English-language bibliography that I have compiled on many aspects of Thai medicine. Nowhere among this material is a complete translation into English of any of the following:

1. The *Tamra phesat* ("Texts on Medicine"), the *Phaetthayasat songkhro* ("The Study of Medicine"), or the *Wetchasu'ksa phaetthayasat sangkhep* ("Manual for Students of Traditional Medicine"): the authoritative texts of Thai herbal education today

2. The Wat Pho massage epigraphs: the famous stone tablets and accompanying inscriptions describing massage techniques
3. Training manuals of the traditional medicine programs at *any* licensed *mo boran* program

The truth is that, without more of these basic translations, or at least more detailed studies on the contents of these texts, we can hardly claim to know much at all about Thai medicine. The few materials that have been translated (by Jean Mulholland for example, who is the only scholar I know to have tackled a complete text, the *Thai Book of Genesis*) show that even the orthodox tradition can be in many respects surprisingly unique.[1]

This ignorance is compounded by the fact that the TTM world remains secretive and reluctant to offer education in translation, with the result that Westerners have yet to participate in the *mo boran* curriculum and licensure system in any significant numbers. Certain elements of Thai medicine, particularly Thai massage, are becoming quite popular both in Thailand and in the West. Short English-language courses in Thai massage designed for tourists have thus opened up all over Chiang Mai and parts of Bangkok. However, the teachers involved in running these schools and courses for the most part are not *mo boran*, but massage technicians with far lesser credentials, and thus the quality of teaching remains on the whole quite low.

Because of the lack of information on Thai massage and TTM more generally, certain misconceptions have arisen that only serve to further obscure Western understanding of these practices. One such problem is a tendency toward absurd claims of antiquity. For example, it is possible to read statements that Thai massage is 2000, 3000, or even 5000 years old. While

---

1 Mulholland (1989). See Bamber (1987) for discussion of another canonical text, the *Prakhampi Krasai*.

the desire for practitioners to posit lengthy lineages for their practices is understandable, these types of statements draw attention away from the fact that Thai medicine, like any medical system, is a living tradition, continuously changing and transforming. As we have seen, hard evidence for Thai massage practice barely extends past the nineteenth century. In fact, there exist no medical writings or other traces of Thai medical culture that extend further back than Ayutthaya, and until such artifacts are discovered, there is no basis whatsoever for making claims that push beyond this threshold.

Another misconception among enthusiasts is that Thai medicine is synonymous with Indian Ayurveda, Chinese medicine, or some combination of the two. A quick search on www. Amazon.com will reveal many books by contemporary teachers and practitioners of Thai massage that make claims that this art is simply applied *hatha-yoga*, or that Thai medicine is interchangeable with Indian Ayurveda. Although throughout this book I have explored connections with other cultures and have even called aspects of Thai medicine "Thai Ayurveda" or "Thai yoga," I strongly advise against thinking of Thai medicine as a corrupted form of another Asian system. This is a mistaken and dangerous view which devalues the tradition and does a disservice to the history of the Thai people.

This critique applies not only to practitioners, but to researchers as well. One approach taken by recent scholarship on Thai medicine has been to lump it together with other Southeast Asian traditions, and to discuss this entire field as an outgrowth of Indian medicine. This approach is flawed because it encourages researchers not to investigate the uniqueness of regional systems and the variations in Southeast Asian medicine across both time and space. In order to better understand local traditions of medicine, we should not just pursue the Indian-influenced material, but also look into the wealth of influences, ideas, and beliefs that characterize the diversity of practices in Southeast Asia while prioritizing the cultural and social factors that determined their appropriation and implementation in each locale.

I hope if I have managed to convey anything in this book it is that we must look at Thai medicine as a diverse and unique tradition. A serious effort needs to be made across different academic and non-academic disciplines in this direction, and dialogue between scholars and practitioners must respect the diversity we will encounter. In these pages, I have explored a number of influences on Thai medicine—from Indian, Chinese, Khmer, T'ai, and Western provenance. However, regardless of the origins of these various elements, it is only in Thailand that this unique synthesis we have been discussing evolved. Traditional Thai medicine today is a syncretic combination of classical healing techniques from across Asia, but it is also a distinctively Thai art. It should be studied as such: not as a branch of Indian or Chinese tradition, but as a vibrant and valuable cultural heritage in its own right.

APPENDICES

APPENDIX A: ANNOTATED BIBLIOGRAPHY OF THAI MEDICAL TEXTS[1]

List of texts on medicine included in the *Phaetthayasat songkhro* ("The Study of Medicine"), with summary of contents:

Volume 1
Phrakhamphi chanthasat
  Eight rules of medical ethics, causes of fever, dysentery, prognosis of death
Phrakhamphi prathomchinda
  Conception, menstruation, the causes of diseases in infants and medicine to treat them
Phrakhamphi thatwiphang
  Abnormalities of the elements according to the seasons
Phrakhamphi sapphakhum
  The properties of drugs

Volume 2
Phrakhamphi samutthanwinitchai
  The search for the cause and origin of disease
Phrakhamphi warayokhasan
  The taste of drugs and characteristics of good and bad omens
Phrakhamphi mahachotarat of Phra-achan Thawsahamobodi Phrom
  Menstruation
Phrakhamphi chawadan
  Food poisoning causing *lom* (air) to aggravate the blood
Phrakhamphi roknithan of Phra-acharn Komaraphat (Jivaka)
  The four *that* (elements) when in excess or deficiency
Phrakhamphi thatwiwon
  The four *that* (elements) and menstruation
Phrakhamphi thatbanchop of Phra-achan Komaraphat (Jivaka)
  Diseases of the bowel caused by the *that* (elements)
Phrakhamphi mutchapakkhantha
  Diseases of the urinary tract and leucorrhea
Phrakhamphi Takkasila
  Complete description of all toxic fevers
Phrakhamphi krasai
  Discussion of a group of diseases of vague causation but producing general weakness and emaciation, 26 types.

1 This information is abridged from Mulholland (1979a), pp. 112-114. Parentheses are mine.

Volume 3
Phrakhamphi aphayasanta
  The origin of fevers and all types of *sang* (congenital defects),
  and diseases of the eyes
Phrakhamphi samutthawinitchai
  See Volume 2.1
Phrakhamphi manchusarawichian
  Diseases of the *lom* (air), 10 types
Phrakhamphi utthararok
  Diseases of dropsy (edema) effecting the abdominal cavity
Phrakhamphi mukkharok
  Diseases of the mouth and throat, 19 types
Phrakhamphi sitthisarasonkhro
  A disease that produces a rash associated with toxic fever or
  toxic inflammation
Phrakhamphi phaichitmahawong
  Abscesses, boils, and pustules
Phrakhamphi thipphamala
  Tuberculosis
Phrakhamphi withikuttaharok
  Leprosy

APPENDIX B: HERBAL MEDICINES BY FLAVOR CATEGORY[2]

Herb	Part	Method	Indications
Astringent			
Rheum palmatum Linn. [Rhubarb]			Nausea, blood in vomit, hemorrhoids, bloody eyes, diarrhea
Rhus verniciflua [Lacquer tree]			Diarrhea, joint pain
Garcinia mangostana [Mangosteen]	Skin		Hemorrhoids
Senna spp.	Bark		Infection of mouth, throat, tooth/gums, general topical cleanser

2 Source: Chaichakan (1997). Information missing from table was not available or missing from original. Brackets [ ] indicate common English name (Thai used when English is unknown or non-existent).

Acacia catechu (Linn. f.) Willd [Catechu]			Diarrhea, topical cleanser
Oroxylum indicum Vent. [Oroxylum]	Bark	Decoction	Diarrhea, chills, post-partum
Tamarindus indica [Tamarind]	Bark	Bath	Topical cleanser
Tamarindus indica [Tamarind]	Pod	Decoction	Diarrhea
Sweet			
Rock sugar		In water	Health, energy, fever, throat
Saccharin		In water	Mucous in throat, emaciation
Sugar		In water	Health, energy, heart, throat
Saccharum spp. [Sugar cane]		In water	Heath, energy, heart, fever, bladder, fatigue, mucous in throat, cough
Brown sugar		In water	Health, energy, fever
Milk			Skin, health
Glycyrrhiza glabra [Licorice]			Throat, mucous, cough
Honey			Asthma, health, longevity
Toxic			
Rheum palmatum Linn. [Rhubarb]			Brain, heart, indigestion, hemorrhoids
Cannabis sativa [Marijuana]			To cause hunger in cases of emaciation. Use small amounts.
Datura metel Linn. [Datura]	Seed	Decoction, Powder, Topical	Fever, rash, ringworm, skin parasites

Entada phaseoloides Merr. [Luk saba]	Seed		Food poisoning, depression
Streblus asper Lour. [Toothbrush tree]		Powder	Ringworm, bone poisoning, muscle, teeth. (Also, can brush teeth with this.)
Diospyros mollis [Ebony tree]	Seed		Tapeworm
Papaver somniferum [Opium]		Smoked	Diarrhea, cough, anesthesia
Phyllanthus acidus Skeels [Star Gooseberry]	Fruit		Swollen lymph nodes, tapeworm, fever
Sulfur		Topical	Skin parasites, mangy dogs.
Bitter			
Tinospora tuberculata Beumee [Heart-leaved moonseed]	Bark		Fever, malaria, lymph, fire element diseases, chronic thirst
Eurycoma longifolia Jack [Tongkat ali]	Root		Food poisoning, persistent cough with fatigue, fever
Sapindus rarak A. DC. [Soap nut]	Seed		Fever, food poisoning
Crocodile	Bile		Bad blood, post-partum, vertigo
Rauvolfia serpentina (L.) Benth. ex Kurz [Rakngayom]	Root		High blood pressure, lymph, worms, intoxicating substitution for cannabis.
Hot			
Piper nigrum [Black pepper]	Fruit		Flatulence, mucous in throat, paralysis
Plumbago zelyanica Linn [Leadwort],	Root		Stimulating digestion, warming the body, stimulating fire element

Plumbago rosea Linn [Rose leadwort]	Bark		Bad blood, amenorrhea
Piper sarmentosum [Wild pepper]	Bark		Mucous, congested lungs, flatulence, indigestion
Moringa oleifera Lom. [Horseradish tree]	Bark		Flatulence, indigestion
Ferula foetida [Asafoetida]			Flatulence, indigestion, mucous, brain
Acorus calamus Linn. [Calamus]	Rhizome		Flatulence, indigestion, water element. Also apply topically to broken bones.
Syzygium aromaticum [Cloves]	Flower	Decoction	Stomach ache, flatulence, frostnip, lymph, uterus, toothache
Ocymum sanctum [Holy basil]	Leaf/root	Decoction	Stomach ache, nausea, promote digestion
Oily			
Sesamum indicum [Sesame]	Seed	Eat	Health, joints, body warmth. (Also, leaves can be steamed and wrapped around sugar and coconut.)
Nuts		Eat	Body warmth, muscle, joints, health, energy.
Castanospormum australe [Black bean]		Eat	Joints, body warmth
Green lentils		Eat	Joints, body warmth
Anacardium occidental [Cashew]	Nut	Eat	Skin disease, rash, infection, dry skin, bones.
Nelumbo nucifera [Lotus]	Seed	Eat	Muscles, skin, joints. Beneficial for pregnancy.

Artocarpus integri-folia [Jackfruit]	Seed	Eat	Health, longevity
Rice		Eat	Joints, fatigue. Beneficial for pregnancy.
Tamarindus indica [Tamarind]	Seed	Eat	Health, worms
Aromatic			
Mimusops elengi Linn. [Bulletwood]		Decoction	Fever, joints, anger, insanity, heart
Mesua ferrea Linn. [Ironwood]		Decoction	Fever, weakness, fatigue, eyes, high blood pressure
Michelia champaca Linn. [Champak]		Decoction	Fever, heart, fatigue, weakness
Canaga odo-rata Lam. [Ylang-ylang]		Decoction	Health, heart, vertigo
Jasminum spp. [Jasmine]	Flower	Decoction	Pregnancy, heart, fever, blood, mucous, thirst, eyes
Telosma odoratissima		Decoction	Lungs, fever, mucous, blood
Salty			
Salt from the sea		Eat	Eyes, lymph, mucous
Salt from the earth		Eat	Constipation, kidney stones, too much grease in stomach
Water with basic pH		Drink	Cleanse stomach, kidneys, bladder, kidney stones, indigestion
Horseshoe crab	Claw	Eat	Beneficial for children and postpartum women, general health.
Rays/skates	Tail	Eat	Beneficial for children and postpartum women, general health.

Cuttlefish		Eat	Gums, acne, mouth sores
Oyster	Shell	Eat	Take ground shell for kidney stones, flatulence, indigestion.
Sour			
Citrus aurantifolia [Lime]	Juice	Drink	Mucous, blood, cough, skin, acne
Citrus hystix [Kaffir lime]	Juice	Drink	Menstruation, mucous
Tamarindus indica [Tamarind]	Juice	Drink	Blood, constipation, before and during delivery
Bouea mac-rophylla Griff [Gandaria]	Fruit	Eat	Mucous in throat, mouth, blood, constipation, fever
Ananas cososus [Pineapple]	Fruit	Eat	Kidney stones, kidneys, bladder, mucous, uterus
Alum powder [derived from aluminum oxide]		Drink in water	Bladder, eyes, ear infection, apply directly to unhealthy loose teeth
Phyllanthus acidus Skeels [Star Gooseberry]		Eat	Fever, mucous, chicken pox, chronic thirst
Bland			
Neptunia plena [Water mimosa]	Fruit	Eat	Take foam that collects on out-side of skin of fruit for fever, food poisoning.
White vegetables		Eat	Eyes, food poisoning
Coccinia indica Wight & Arn [Ivy gourd]			Food poisoning, purgative
Graptophyllum pictum [Caricature plant]			Fever, chronic thirst, chicken pox, food poisoning
Clay, rich in aluminum		Powder	Apply with water to skin for rashes, overheating.

Thunbergia lauri-folia Linn [Purple Allamanda]	Bark	Decoction	Fever, hang-over
Cordyline fruti-cosa A. Cheval [Ti plant]		Decoction	Gargle with decoction for infected or bleeding gums, bad breath. Drink tea for chicken pox, fever.

APPENDIX C: HERBAL MEDICINES BY SYMPTOM[3]

Herb	Part	Method
Digestion		
Cymbopogon citratus [Lemongrass]	Leaves/stalk	Decoction
Syzygium aromaticum [Cloves]	Flower	Decoction/Powder
Zingiber officinale [Ginger]	Rhizome	Decoction
Allium sativum [Garlic]	Bulb	Food
Languas galanga Sw, Alpinia galanga Stunz [Galanga]	Rhizome	Decoction
Amomum xanthi-oides Wall [Bastard cardamom]	Seed	Powder
Amomum krervanh [Cardamom]	Seed	Decoction/Powder
Gas/Flatulence		
Ocymum sanctum [Holy basil]	Leaves	Decoction
Boesenbergia pandu-rata Holtt [Finger root]	Rhizome	Decoction

3   Source: Chaichakan (1997).

Zingiber zerumbet Rosc. Smith [Zerumbet ginger]	Rhizome	Decoction
Piper Sylvaticum	Flower	Decoction
Cyperus rotundus Linn. [Ya heawmoo]	Root	Decoction
Citrus aurantifolia [Lime]	Skin	Decoction, or add to curry
Fever		
Tinospora tuberculata Beumee [Heart-leaved moonseed]	Stalk	Decoction
Eurycoma longifolia Jack [Tongkat ali]	Root	Decoction, drink morning and evening
Andrographis paniculata [Chiretta]	Stalk/leaves	Decoction (also stalk can be chewed for toothache)
Tiliacora triandra Diels [Yanang]	Root	Decoction, drink 3 times daily
Skin Infections		
Cassia alata Linn [Candelabra bush]	Leaves	Apply topically
Allium sativum [Garlic]	Bulb	Apply topically
Rhinacanthus nasutus (L.) Kurz [Thong phan chang]	Root/leaves/stalk	Tincture in alcohol
Languas galanga Sw, Alpinia galanga Stunz [Galanga]	Rhizome	Tincture in alcohol
Diarrhea		
Punica granatum [Pomegranate]	Skin (dried)	Decoction, or eat with water and slaked lime

Garcinia mangostana [Mangosteen]	Skin (dried)	Decoction
Tamarindus indica [Tamarind]	Bark	Decoction
Mesua sapientum [Banana]	Fruit	Eat unripe
Acacia catechu (Linn. f.) Willd [Catechu]	Sap	1 tsp., boiled in water
Psidium guajava [Guava]	Leaf	Decoction from 10 flame-roasted leaves, or mash unripe fruit in water, drink
Sesbania grandi-flora (Desv.) Linn. [Corkwood tree]	Bark	Decoction from flame-roasted bark
Constipation		
Senna spp.	Leaves	Decoction or powder (especially beneficial for elderly)
Cassia alata Linn. [Candelabra bush]	Flowers/leaves	Eat fresh flowers, or make tea from leaves
Cassia fistula Linn. [Golden shower]	Seed	Boil with salt and eat
Bridelia burmanica [MaKa]	Leaves	Roast 15 leaves, decoct with salt and drink in morning or before sleep
Tamarindus indica [Tamarind]	Fruit	Eat
Cassia siamea Lamk. [Siamese cassia]	Stalk	Decoction before meal and/or before sleep.
Cassia tora Linn. [Foetid cassia]	Seed	Decoction from dry-roast dried seed

Tapeworm		
Diospyros mollis [Ebony tree]	Fruit	Mash fresh fruit with coconut milk and drink. Adult dosage: 25 fruits, children:1 fruit for each year of age. Do not use with children under 10
Artocarpus lakoocha Roxb. [Monkey jack]	Pod	Boil pod, collect foam on top, make powder, mix 1 tsp with cold water. (Don't use warm water to avoid nausea.) Take before meals.
Combretum quad-rangulare Kurz [Combretum]	Seed	Grind finely, eat 1 tsp on fried eggs.
Curbita spp. [Pumpkin]	Seed	Grind 60 g in 500 cc water. Drink 3x at 2 hour intervals.
Tamarindus indica [Tamarind]	Seed	Dry roast 30 seeds, soak in water until soft. Eat.
Punica granatum [Pomegranate]	Bark of tree or skin of root	Decoction, taken in morning. (May cause headache or nausea.)
Quisqualis indica Linn. [Rangoon creeper]	Seed	Decoction. Adult dosage: 5-7, children: 2-3.
Nausea/Vomiting		
Ocymum sanctum [Holy basil]	Leaf	Decoction
Zingiber officinale [Ginger]	Rhizome	Decoction
Piper sylvaticum	Flower or fruit	Decoction

Cymbopogon citratus [Lemongrass]	Stalk	Decoction
Morinda citrifolia Linn. [Indian mulberry]	Fruit	Decoction from 2 handfuls of flame-roasted fruits.
Food Poisoning/Hives		
Garcinia mangostana [Mangosteen]	Skin	Powder from flame-roasted skin. Drink with hot water.
Acacia catechu (Linn. f.) Willd [Catechu]	Wood	Boil to make a thick paste. Take 1/2 tsp in hot water.
Boesenbergia pandu-rata Holtt [Finger root]	Root	Decoct from root, fresh and flame-roasted, or dried.
Zingiber zerumbet Rosc. Smith [Zerumbet ginger]	Rhizome	Flame roast and decoct.
Punica granatum [Pomegranate]	Skin of fruit	Decoction

Annotated Bibliography of Thai Language Sources[1]

Ayurawet Withayalai. *Tamra Kanphaetthaidoem – Phaetsatsongkhro (Text of Original Thai Medicine – Compilation of Medicine)*. Bangkok: Rongpim SiThai, 1998. This is a summary of the original texts of Thai Medicine compiled by King Rama the Fifth, *Phaetsatsongkhro*. This particular version is from the Ayurawet University.

Darot, Mathayat. *Naenaeokansopwicha Wet-Phesachakampaenboran (Guidelines for examination in Medical Theory and Pharmacy)*. Bangkok: Mathayat, 1977. One of the most commonly used books to aid in the study of Thai Traditional Medicine. It includes summaries of both pharmacy and medical theory.

Faculty of Pharmacy at Mahidol University. *Samunphrai Suan Sirirukkhachat (Herbal Plants at Sirirukkhachat Garden)*. Bangkok: Amarin Printing Group, 1992. Contains very clear pictures of the medicinal plants at the garden. It also includes a description of the plant along with uses.

Faculty of Pharmacy at Mahidol University. *Sapphaetthai (Terminology of Thai Medicine)*. Bangkok: Prachachon Chamkat, 1994. Includes a list of all major texts from which the terms explained in the book are taken. Included are page numbers and volumes. This is one of the most useful books to help understand TTM.

Ministry of Education. *Mothai Yathai (Thai Doctors, Thai Medicine)*. Bangkok: National Identity Dissemination Project, 1978. One of the most practical and comprehensive books on Thai Medicine of the past. It includes essays written by various traditional doctors. Included is a thorough explanation of diagnosis in Thai Medicine.

Ministry of Education. *Tamra Charuek Wat Raja Orot lae Phra Osot Phra Narai (Textbook of Inscriptions from Raja Osot Temple and Phra Osot Phra Narai's Manual)*. Bangkok: National Dissemination Project, 1978. Contains transcriptions

---

1 This bibliography is included courtesy of Wit Sukhsamran.

and translations, into modern Thai, of the inscriptions located at Raja Osot Temple. Included is information about both massage and herbal medicine.

Phichiansunton, Chayan, Chawalit, Maenamat and Chiruang, Wichian. *Kamathibai Tamra Phra Osoth Phra Narai (Explanation of the Text of Phra Osoth Phra Narai).* Bangkok: Samnakphim Amarin, 2001. Explains the oldest and only text remaining from the Ayuthaya period on Thai Traditional Medicine. It contains detailed explanations of the formulas and theory contained within this ancient text.

Phrayaphisanuprasatwet, School of The Medical Society. *Vechasueksapaetsatsangk hep Lem 1-3 (A Summary of the Study of Medical Theory, Books 1-3).* Bangkok: Phaisansin Kanphim, 1988. One version of the summary of medical theory collected and compiled by King Rama the Fifth.

Pongphamon, Pricha. *Tamra Yaphaetphaenboran (Textbook of Traditional Medicine).* Bangkok: Amnuaisan, 1979. Includes not only descriptions of the most commonly used herbs in Thai formulas, but also has over 100 formulas for various ailments. The formulas included in this book are still used quite frequently today.

Prasoet, Nai and the Faculty of Traditional Medicine at Wat Maha That. *Tamra Phesachakamthaiphaenboran (The Textbook of Thai Traditional Pharmacy).* Bangkok: Mahachulalongkron Rachawithayalai, 1988. This book is a rare find. It is from the Traditional School of Medicine at Wat Maha That. At one time this was a thriving school for medicine. This book covers the curriculum at the school.

Sapcharoen, Phennapha. *Kanphaetphaenthai Kanpaetbaepongruam (Methods of Thai Medicine and its Uses).* Nonthaburi: Foundation for Thai Traditional Medicine, 1996. This book gives a summary of what Thai medicine is and how it is used. It is one of the most popular books among the general public on the topic.

School of Traditional Medicine at Wat Phra Chetuphon. *Wechasueksa (The Study of Medicine).* Bangkok: Mahamakutrachavithayalai, 1963. This is one of the texts from Wat Pho on Thai Traditional Medical Theory. It is one of the oldest modern texts and has been referenced in most, if not all, books and texts used in schools today.

School of Traditional Medicine at Wat Phra Chetuphon. *Paetsatsongkhro Lem 1 (The Compilation of Medicine Book 1).* Bangkok: Phaisan, 1963; *Book 2,* 1963; *Book 3,* 1963. The Wat Pho version of King Rama V's collection of knowledge on Thai Traditional Medicine. Again, these books have been referenced in most, if not all, books and texts used in schools today.

School of Traditional Medicine at Wat Phra Chetuphon. *Phramuan Sapakunyathai*

Lem 1 (A Collection of the Properties of Medicine Book 1). Bangkok: Mahama kutrachavithayalai, 1964; *Book 2*, 1973; *Book 3*, 1977. This is a collection of names, characteristics, properties and uses of many of the plants used in the Thai materia medica.

School of Traditional Medicine at Wat Phra Chetuphon. *Tamra Pramuanlakphesat (The Textbook on the Codification of the Pillars of Pharmacy)*. Bangkok: Sithai, 1985. This book from Wat Pho is used as the primary text for the pharmacy curriculum.

Social Research Institute at Chiang Mai University. *Tamra Samunphrailanna (Textbook of Northern Herbs)*. Chiang Mai: Chiang Mai University, 1982. This is one of the few books published which includes traditional medicine formulas from North Thailand. Some formulas are similar to those found in other areas of the country, but most are unique to the North.

Thiangbunnatham, Wit. *Phochanukrom Roklaesamunphraithai (Dictionary of Disease and Thai Herbs)*. Bangkok: Rongphim Aksonphithaya, 1990. This is a dictionary of various diseases and herbal formulas used to treat those diseases.

Thiangbunnatham, Wit. *Phochanukrom Samunphraithai (Dictionary of Thai Herbs)*. Bangkok: Rongphim Aksonphithaya, 1990. A listing of over 500 Thai Herbs with botanical names and descriptions. Included is a list of uses and some hand drawn illustrations.

Wuthithammawet, Wuth. *Khamphiphesatratanakosin (Treatise of Pharmacy of the Current Era)*. Bangkok: Wuthikammawet, 2004. A collection of information needed for the study of Thai traditional pharmacy. Included is a section on the properties of many of the drugs used in the Thai pharmacopia.

Wuthithammawet, Wuth. *Saranukromsamunphrai (Encyclopedia of Herbs)*. Bangkok: Odian Store, 1995. This is one of the most thorough collections of the Thai materia medica. It includes pictures, descriptions and properties of over a thousand different drugs; plant, animal and mineral.

Bibliography of English Language Sources

Anderson, Edward F. *Plants and People of the Golden Triangle: Ethnobotany of the Hill Tribes of Northern Thailand.* Portland, Ore: Dioscorides Press, 1993.

Anusaranashasanakiarti, Phra Khru. "Funerary Rites and the Buddhist Meaning of Death: An Interpretative Text from Northern Thailand." In *Journal of the Siam Society,* 68:1(1980):1-28.

Attagara, Kingkeo. *The Folk Religion of Ban Nai, A Hamlet in Central Thailand.* Diss. Ph.D., Indiana University, 1967.

Aymonier, Etienne. *Khmer Heritage in Thailand with Special Emphasis on Temples, Inscriptions and Etymology.* Bangkok: White Lotus Press, 1999. (Reprint from 1901.)

Bamber, Scott. "Metaphor and Illness Classification in Traditional Thai Medicine." In *Asian Folklore Studies* 46:2(1987):179-95.

Bamber, Scott. "Medicine, Food, and Poison in Traditional Thai Healing." In Morris F. Low, ed., *Beyond Joseph Needham: Science, Technology and Medicine in East and Southeast Asia. Osiris,* 13(1998):339-353.

Blimes, Jack. "The Individual and His Environment: A Central Thai Outlook." In *Journal of the Siam Society,* 65(1977):2:153-162.

Boesch, Ernst E. *Communication Between Doctors and Patients in Thailand, Part I: Survey of the Problem and Analysis of the Consultations.* Saarbrücken, Germany: University of the Saar, 1972.

Boisselier, Jean. *Thai Painting.* Tokyo, New York and San Francisco: Kodansha International, 1976.

Bowen, John R. "The Forms Culture Takes: A State-of-the-Field Essay on the Anthropology of Southeast Asia." In *The Journal of Asian Studies* 54:4(1995):1047-1078.

Bradley, Dan Beach. "Siamese Practice of Medicine." In *Bangkok Calendar,* 1865. Reprinted in *Sangkhomsat Parithat,* 5:3(1967):83-94.

Bragg, Katherine. "The Akha: Folk Botany and Forest Traditions." In Walton, Geoffrey, *A Northern Miscellany: Essays from the North of Thailand.* Chiang Mai and Bangkok: Silkworm Books, 1992.

Traditional Thai Medicine

Brown, Robert, ed. *Art From Thailand*. Mumbai: Marg, 1999.

Brun, Viggo, and Trond Schumacher, *Traditional Herbal Medicine in Northern Thailand*, Berkeley and Los Angeles: University of California Press, 1987. Reprint: Bangkok, White Lotus Co., 1994.

Brun, Viggo. "Traditional Thai Medicine." In Helaine Selin and Hugh Shapiro, eds. *Medicine Across Cultures: History and Practice of Medicine in Non-Western Cultures*. Boston and London: Kluwer Academic Publishers, 2003.

Chaichakan Sintorn. *Traditional Medicine Hospital Handbook for Course in Thai Medicine*. Chiang Mai: Shivagakomarpaj Traditional Medicine Hospital, 1997.

Chhem, Kieth Rethy. "A Khmer Medical Text 'The Treatment of the Four Diseases' Manuscript." In *Journal of the Center for Khmer Studies*, 6(2004):33-42.

Chirapravati, ML Pattaratorn. *Votive Tablets in Thailand: Origin, Style, and Uses*. Kuala Lumpur and New York: Oxford University Press, 1997.

Chokevivat, Vichai, et al. "The Use of Traditional Medicine in the Thai Health Care System." World Health Organization Regional Office for South-East Asia: Regional Consultation on Development of Traditional Medicine in the South East Asia Region, Pyongyang, DPR Korea, 22-24 June, 2005. Document no. 9.

Chokevivat, Vichai, and Anchalee Chuthaputti. "The Role of Thai Traditional Medicine in Health Promotion." Department for the Development of Thai Traditional and Alternative Medicine, Ministry of Public Health, 6GCHP Bangkok Thailand 7-11 Aug, 2005.

Coedès, G. *The Making of South East Asia*. Berkeley and Los Angeles: University of California Press, 1966.

Coedès, G. *The Indianized States of Southeast Asia*. Honolulu: East-West Center Press, 1968.

Coughlin, Richard J. *Double Identity: The Chinese in Modern Thailand*. Hong Kong: Hong Kong University Press, 1960.

Dash, Vaidya Bhagwan. *Materia Medica of Ayurveda: Based on Mandanapala's Nighantu*. New Delhi: B. Jain Publishers, 1991.

de la Loubère, Simon. *The Kingdom of Siam*. London and New York: Oxford University Press, 1969. (Reprint from 1693 English edition.)

Demiéville, Paul. "Byo." In Sylvain Lévi et al., eds., *Hobogirin dictionnaire encyclopédique du bouddhisme d'après les sources chinoises et japonaises*. Tokyo: Maison Franco-Japonaise, 1929. Reprinted in translation in Mark Tatz ed., *Buddhism and Healing: Demiéville's Article "Byo" from Hobogirin*. Lanham, MD: University Press of America, 1985.

References

Fadiman, Ann. *The Spirit Catches You and You Fall Down*. New York: Farrar, Straus and Giroux, 1998.

Feuerstein, Georg. *The Yoga Tradition: Its History, Literature, Philosophy, and Practice*. Prescott, Ariz.: Hohm Press, 2001.

Fisher, Robert E. *Buddhist Art and Architecture*. London and New York: Thames & Hudson, 1993.

Flood, Gavin. *An Introduction to Hinduism*. Cambridge University Press, 1996.

Formoso, Bernard, "Hsiu-Hou-Ku: The Ritual Refining of Restless Ghosts Among the Chinese of Thailand." In *Journal of the Royal Anthropological Institute*, 2:2(1996):217-234.

Frawley, David. *Yoga & Ayurveda: Self-Healing and Self-Realization*. Twin Lakes, Wisc.: Lotus Press, 1999.

Golomb, Louis. *An Anthropology of Curing in Multiethnic Thailand*. Urbana and Chicago: University of Illinois Press, 1985.

Golomb, Louis. "Supernaturalist Cures and Sorcery Accusations in Thailand." In *Soc. Sci. Med.*, 27:5(1988):437-443.

Golomb, Louis. "The Relevancy of Magical Malevolence in Urban Thailand." In C.W. Watson and Roy Ellen, eds. *Understanding Witchcraft and Sorcery in Southeast Asia*. Honolulu: University of Hawaii Press, 1993.

Gosling, David. "Thailand's Bare-Headed Doctors." In *Modern Asian Studies* 19:4(1985):761-796.

Griswold, A. B. "The Rishis of Wat Po." In *Felicitation Volumes of Southeast-Asian Studies Presented to His Highness Prince Dhaninivat Kromamun Bidyalabh Brindhyakorn*. Bangkok: The Siam Society, 1965.

Griswold, A. B. and Prasert Na Nagara. "On Kingship and Society at Sukothai." In Skinner, G. William and A. Thomas Kirsch, eds., *Change and Persistence in Thai Society: Essays in Honor of Lauriston Sharp*. Ithaca and London: Cornell University Press, 1975, p. 29-92.

Harper, Donald. "A Chinese Demonography of the Third Century B.C." In *Harvard Journal of Asiatic Studies* 45:2(1985):459-98.

Hawkes, David, trans. *The Songs of the South: an Ancient Chinese Anthology of Poems by Qu Yuan and Other Poets*. New York: Penguin Books, 1985.

Heinze, Ruth-Inge. "Nature and Function of Some Therapeutic Techniques in Thailand." In *Asian Folklore Studies*, 2(1977):85-104.

Heinze, Ruth-Inge. *Tham Khwan: How to Contain the Essence of Life, A Socio-Psychological Comparison of a Thai Custom*. Singapore: Singapore University Press, 1982.

Heinze, Ruth-Inge. "The Relationship Between Folk and Elite Religions: The Case of Thailand." In Sitakant Mahapatra, ed. *The Realm of the Sacred: Verbal Symbolism and Ritual Structures*. Calcutta: Oxford University Press, 1992.

Heinze, Ruth-Inge. *Trance and Healing in Southeast Asia Today, Second edition*. Bangkok: White Lotus Press, 1997.

Hill, Ann Maxwell. "Chinese Funerals and Chinese Ethnicity in Chiang Mai, Thailand." In *Ethnology*, 31:4(1992):315-30.

Hinderling, Paul. *Communication between Doctors and Patients in Thailand: A Report from the South Asia Research Programme (Part III: Interviews with Traditional Doctors)*. Saarbrücken, Germany: University of the Saar, 1973.

Hodges, Ian. "Western Science in Siam: A Tale of Two Kings." In Morris F. Low, ed., *Beyond Joseph Needham: Science, Technology and Medicine in East and Southeast Asia*. Osiris 13(1998):80-95.

Hofbauer, Rudolf. "A Medical Retrospect of Thailand." In *Journal of the Thailand Research Society*, 34(1943):183-200.

Horner, I.B. *The Book of the Discipline (Vinaya-Pitaka)* Vol. IV. Oxford: Pali Text Society, 2000.

Jacquat, Christiane. *Plants from the Markets of Thailand*. Bangkok: Editions Duang Kamol, 1990.

Kenjiro, Ichikawa, "The Assimilation of Chinese in Changing Thai Society." In *Japanese Journal of Ethnology*, 31:4(1967):277-280.

Kirch, A. Thomas. "Complexity in the Thai Religious System: An Interpretation." In *Journal of Asian Studies*, 36:2(1977):241-266.

Kleinman, Arthur. *Patients and Healers in the Context of Culture*. Berkeley: University of California, 1980.

Krairiksh, Piriya. *The Sacred Image: Sculptures from Thailand*. Cologne: Museen der Stadt Köln, 1979-1980.

Lamotte, Étienne. *History of Indian Buddhism: From the Origins to the Shaka Era*. Louvain and Paris: Peeters Press, 1988. (Reprint from 1958.)

Le May, Reginald. *The Culture of South-East Asia: The Heritage of India*. London: George Allen & Unwin Ltd., 1964.

Lockard, Craig A. "Integrating Southeast Asia into the Framework of World History: The Period Before 1500," in *The History Teacher*, 29:1(1995):7-35.

Lord, D.C. *Mo Bradley and Thailand*. Grand Rapids: W. Eerdmans, 1969.

Matics, K.I. "Medical Arts at Wat Phra Chetuphon: Various Rishi Statues." In *Journal of the Siam Society*, 65:2(1977):145-152.

References

Matics, K.I. *An Historical Analysis of the Fine Arts at Wat Phra Chetuphon: A Repository of Ratanakosin Artistic Heritage.* Diss. Ph.D., New York University, 1978.

Matics, K.I. *A History of Wat Phra Chetuphon and its Buddha Images.* Bangkok: Siam Society, 1979.

Matics, K.I. "Major Buddhist Images at Wat Po." In *Arts of Asia*, 12(Nov-Dec 1982):96-103.

McFarland, George Bradley. *Thai English Dictionary.* Stanford: Stanford University Press, 1944.

McMakin, Patrick D. *Flowering Plants of Thailand: A Field Guide.* Bangkok: White Lotus Co., 2000.

Menakanit, Alisara. *A Royal Temple in the Thai Urban Landscape: Wat Pho, Bangkok.* Diss. Ph.D., Texas A&M University, 1999.

Ministry of Commerce and Communications. *Some Siamese Medicinal Plants exhibited at the Eighth Congress of Far Eastern Association of Tropical Medicine.* Bangkok: Ministry of Commerce and Communications, Botanical Section, 1930.

Mulholland, Jean. "Thai Traditional Medicine: Ancient Thought and Practice in a Thai Context." In *Journal of the Siam Society*, 67:2(1979a):80-115.

Mulholland, Jean. "Thai Traditional Medicine—The Treatment of Diseases Caused by the Tridosha." In *The South East Asian Review*, 3:2(1979b):29-38.

Mulholland, Jean. "Traditional Medicine in Thailand." In *Hemisphere*, 23:4(July/Aug 1979c):224-229.

Mulholland, Jean. *Medicine, Magic, and Evil Spirits.* Canberra: Australian National University, 1987.

Mulholland, Jean. "Ayurveda, Congenital Disease and Birthdays in Thai Traditional Medicine." In *Journal of the Siam Society*, 76(1988):174-182.

Mulholland, Jean. *Herbal Medicine in Paediatrics: Translation of a Thai Book of Genesis.* Canberra: Australian National University, 1989.

National Identity Board. *Medicinal Plants of Thailand Past and Present.* Bangkok: National Identity Board, 1991.

Nivat, H.H. Prince Dhani. "The Inscriptions of Wat Phra Jetubon." In *Journal of the Siam Society*, 26:2(1933):143-170.

Pecharaply, Daroon. *Indigenous Medicinal Plants of Thailand.* Bangkok: Department of Medical Sciences, Ministry of Public Health, 1994.

Rajadhon, Phya Anuman. "The Khwan and its Ceremonies." In *Journal of the Siam Society*, 50(1962):119-164.

Rajadhon, Phya Anuman. "Thai Charms and Amulets." In *Journal of the Siam Society*, 52(1964):171-197.

Rajadhon, Phya Anuman. "Data on Conditioned Poison (A Folklore Study)." In *Journal of the Siam Society*, 53:1(1965):69-82.

Ratarasarn, Somchintana Thongthew. *The Socio-cultural Setting of Love Magic in Central Thailand*. Madison: University of Wisconsin Center for Southeast Asian Studies, 1979.

Ratarasarn, Somchintana. *The Principles and Concepts of Thai Classical Medicine*. Bangkok: Thai Khadi Research Institute, Thammasat University, 1989.

Research and Development Institute, Government Pharmaceutical Organization, *www.rdi.gpo.or.th*, accessed Jun. to Aug., 2001.

Reynolds, Frank E. and Mari B. *Three Worlds According to King Ruang: A Thai Buddhist Cosmology*. Berkeley: Asian Humanities Press, 1982.

Reynolds, Frank. "Civic Religion and National Community in Thailand." In *Journal of Asian Studies*, 36:2(1977):267-283.

Saddhatissa, Ven. Dr., and Maurice Walshe, trans. *Chanting Book: Morning and Evening Puja and Reflections*. Hertfordshire (UK): Amaravati Publications, 1994.

Saralamp, Promjit, et al. *Medicinal Plants in Thailand, Vol. 1-2*. Bangkok: Department of Pharmaceutical Botany, Mahidol University, 1996-1997.

Skinner, G. William. *Chinese Society in Thailand: An Analytical History*. Ithaca and New York: Cornell University Press, 1957.

Skinner, G. William and Thomas Kirsch. *Change and Persistence in Thai Society: Essays in Honor of Lauriston Sharp*. Ithaca and London: Cornell University Press, 1975.

Strickmann, Michel. *Chinese Magical Medicine*. Stanford: Stanford University Press, 2002.

Suwanlert, Sangun. "*Phii Pob*: Spirit Possession in Rural Thailand." In William P. Lebra, ed. *Culture-Bound Syndromes, Ethnopsychiatry, and Alternate Therapies: Volume IV of Mental Health Research in Asia and the Pacific*. Honolulu: University of Hawaii Press, 1976.

Tambiah, Stanley Jeyaraja. *Buddhism and the Spirit Cults in North-East Thailand*. Cambridge: Cambridge University Press, 1970.

Tambiah, Stanley Jeyaraja. *World Conqueror and World Renouncer: A Study of Buddhism and Polity in Thailand against a Historical Background*. Cambridge: Cambridge University Press, 1976.

Tambiah, Stanley Jeyaraja. "The Cosmological and Performative Significance

References

of a Thai Cult of Healing Through Meditation." In *Culture, Medicine and Psychiatry*, 1(1977):97-132.

Tambiah, Stanley Jeyaraja. *The Buddhist Saints of the Forest and the Cult of Amulets.* Cambridge: Cambridge University Press, 1984.

Tannenbaum, Nicola. "Witches, Fortune, and Misfortune among the Shan of Northwestern Thailand." In C.W. Watson and Roy Ellen, eds. *Understanding Witchcraft and Sorcery in Southeast Asia.* Honolulu: University of Hawaii Press, 1993.

Tarling, Nicholas, ed. *The Cambridge History of Southeast Asia.* New York: Cambridge University Press, 1992.

Techatraisak, Bongkotrat. *Traditional Medical Practitioners in Bangkok: A Geographical Analysis.* Diss. Ph.D., University of North Carolina, Chapel Hill, 1985.

Terwiel, B.J. "A Model for the Study of Thai Buddhism." In *Journal of Asian Studies*, 35:3(1976):391-403.

Terwiel, B.J. "The Origin of the T'ai Peoples Reconsidered." In *Oriens Extremus*, 25:2(1978a):239-259.

Terwiel, B.J. "The T'ais and Their Belief in Khwans: Towards Establishing an Aspect of 'Proto-T'ai' Culture." In *The South East Asian Review*, 3:1(1978b):1-16.

Terwiel, B.J. *A History of Modern Thailand 1767-1942.* St. Lucia, London and New York: University of Queensland Press, 1983.

Terwiel, B.J. *Monks and Magic: An Analysis of Religious Ceremonies in Central Thailand.* Bangkok and Cheney: White Lotus Press, 1994.

Textor, Robert B. *An Inventory of Non-Buddhist Supernatural Objects in a Central Thai Village.* Diss. Ph.D., Cornell University, 1960.

Thai Pharmaceutical Committee. *Thai Herbal Pharmacopoeia.* Bangkok: Department of Medical Sciences, Ministry of Public Health, 1995.

Van Esterik, Penny. "To Strengthen and Refresh: Herbal Therapy in Southeast Asia." In *Soc. Sci. Med.* 27:8(1988):751-759.

Wales, H.G. Quaritch. "Siamese Theory and Ritual Connected with Pregnancy, Birth and Infancy." In *Journal of the Royal Anthropological Institute of Great Britain and Ireland*, 63(Jul.-Dec., 1933):441-451.

Wales, H.G. Quaritch. *The Universe Around Them: Cosmology and Cosmic Renewal in Indianized South-east Asia.* London: Arthur Probsthain, 1977.

Wales, H.G. Quaritch. *Divination in Thailand: The Hopes and Fears of a Southeast Asian People.* London and Dublin: Curzon Press, 1981.

Wibulbolprasert, Suwit, ed. *Thailand Health Profile 2001-2004.* Nonthaburi: Bureau of Policy and Strategy, Ministry of Public Health, 2005.

Wright, Michael A. "Some Observations on Thai Animism." In *Practical Anthropology*, 15(1968):1-7.

Wujastyk, Dominik. *The Roots of Ayurveda*. London: Penguin Books, 2003.

Zysk, Kenneth G. "Studies in Traditional Indian Medicine in the Pali Canon: Jivaka and *Ayurveda*." In *Journal of the International Association of Buddhist Studies*, 5:1(1982):70-86.

Zysk, Kenneth G. *Religious Medicine: The History and Evolution of Indian Medicine*. New Brunswick and London: Transaction Publishers, 1993a. (Reprint of 1985 original.)

Zysk, Kenneth G. "The Science of Respiration and the Doctrine of the Bodily Winds in Ancient India." In *Journal of the American Oriental Society* 113:2(1993b):198-213.

Zysk, Kenneth G. *Asceticism and Healing in Ancient India: Medicine in the Buddhist Monastery*. Delhi: Motilal Banarsidass, 1998. (Reprint of 1991 original.)

Zysk, Kenneth G. "New Age Ayurveda, or What Happens to Indian Medicine When it Comes to America." In *Traditional South Asian Medicine*, 6(2001):10-26.

Index

Index

Other Titles of Interest from Hohm Press

THE YOGA TRADITION: *Its History, Literature, Philosophy and Practice*
by Georg Feuerstein, Ph.D.

A complete overview of the great Yogic traditions of: Raja-Yoga, Hatha-Yoga, Jnana-Yoga, Bhakti-Yoga, Karma-Yoga, Tantra-Yoga, Kundalini-Yoga, Mantra-Yoga and many other lesser known forms. Includes translations of over twenty famous Yoga treatises, like the *Yoga-Sutra* of Patanjali, and a first-time translation of the *Goraksha Paddhati*, an ancient Hatha Yoga text. Covers all aspects of Hindu, Buddhist, Jaina and Sikh Yoga. A necessary resource for all students and scholars of Yoga.

Paper, 540 pages, over 200 illustrations, $29.95. ISBN: 1-890772-18-6.

KISHIDO: *The Way of the Western Warrior*
by Peter Hobart

The code of the samurai and the path of the knight-warrior, traditions from opposite sides of the globe, find a common ground in *Kishido: the Way of the Western Warrior*. In fifty short essays, Peter Hobart presents the wisdom, philosophy and teachings of the mysterious Master who first united the noble houses of East and West. Kishido prioritizes the ideals of duty, ethics, courtesy and chivalry, from whatever source they derive. This cross-cultural approach represents a return to time-honored principles from many traditions, and allows the modern reader from virtually any background to find the master within.

Paper, 130 pages, $12.95   ISBN: 1-890772-31-3

To order: 1-800-381-2700 or visit our website www.hohmpress.com

JOURNEY TO HEAVENLY MOUNTAIN: An American's Pilgrimage to the Heart of Buddhism in Modern China
by Jay Martin

"I came to China to live in Buddhist monasteries and to revisit my soul," writes best-selling American author and distinguished scholar Jay Martin of his 1998 pilgrimage. This book is an account of one man's spiritual journey. His intention? To penetrate the soul of China and its wisdom. *Journey to Heavenly Mountain* is about the author's desire to know God and sacred things. It is about his yearning for illuminated insight and his hunger to achieve virtue and calmness of spirit. Martin focuses on the profound richness and varieties of inner life, along with the potential for growth in wisdom and empathy which life among these dedicated Buddhists offered.

"Well-written and intelligent, it will appeal to both casual readers and to specialists." —Library Journal

Paper, 264 pages, 12 photos, $16.95   ISBN: 1-890772-17-8

BEYOND ASPIRIN: Nature's Challenge To Arthritis, Cancer & Alzheimer's Disease
by Thomas A. Newmark and Paul Schulick

A reader-friendly guide to one of the most remarkable medical breakthroughs of our times. Research shows that inhibition of the COX-2 enzyme significantly reduces the inflammation that is currently linked with arthritis, colon and other cancers, and Alzheimer's disease. Challenging the conventional pharmaceutical "silver-bullet" approach, this book pleads a convincing case for the safe and effective use of the COX-2-inhibiting herbs, including green tea, rosemary, basil, ginger, turmeric and others.

Paper, 340 pages, $14.95   ISBN: 0-934252-82-3
Cloth; 340 pages, $24.95   ISBN: 1-890772-01-1

136

GINGER: Common Spice & Wonder Drug (Third Edition)
by Paul Schulick

For thousands of years ginger has been one of the world's most favored spices and a major ingredient in Oriental remedies. Yet, ginger's precious healing values are still virtually unknown and ignored in the modern world. This book proposes that ginger is a healing substance beyond the therapeutic scope of any modern drug; a substance with the potential to save billions of dollars and countless lives. Supported by hundreds of scientific studies, this book leads the reader to discover the extraordinary personal and social benefits of using ginger.

"A wonderful collection of information. A convincing case."
—Andrew Weil, M.D., best-selling author of *Spontaneous Healing*

Paper; $9.95, 176 pages   ISBN: 1-890772-07-0

THE DETOX MIRACLE SOURCEBOOK
Raw Food and Herbs for Complete Cellular Regeneration
by Robert S. Morse, N.D.

"You don't have to accept the 'death sentence' offered by other medical systems," Dr. Morse has told thousands of patients over the years. Since 1972, he has directed a health clinic in Florida, successfully helping people cure themselves of cancer, diabetes, M.S., Crohn's disease, along with both brain and nerve damage. His "miracle" approach is fully detailed in this comprehensive book. Morse's system is to treat the cause of illness, not the symptoms! It shows you how to use raw foods and herbs as the primary means of detoxification, healing, and ultimate regeneration of weak or diseased cells.

Paper, $29.95, 384 pages   ISBN: 1-890772-33-X

TRAVEL HEALTHY
A Guidebook for Health-Conscious Travelers
by Lalitha Thomas

This book will "go" anywhere, whether your itinerary calls for a day trip to your local state park or an odyssey around the world. Lalitha Thomas, author of the highly-acclaimed *Ten Essential Herbs* and *Ten Essential Foods*, will show you how to prepare a Health-Smart Travel Kit, and how to use it! You'll learn how to apply natural and healthy means to prevent and to remedy dozens of minor emergencies and major inconveniences, like: indigestion ... food poisoning ... jet lag ... poor water ... poor air ... colds and flus ... toothache ... diarrhea ... constipation ... pesky insects, including bedbugs ... sunburn ... and more.

Lalitha has traveled with children throughout Mexico, India and Europe. Each chapter contains a section of *Tips for Kids*—simple ways to make their trip more enjoyable and to help them stay healthy on the road, in the air, or on the water.

Paper, $9.95, 120 pages   ISBN: 1-890772-25-9

ZEN TRASH
The Irreverent and Sacred Teaching Stories of Lee Lozowick
Edited and with Commentary by Sylvan Incao

This book contains dozens of teaching stories from many world religious traditions — including Zen, Christianity, Tibetan Buddhism, Sufism and Hinduism — rendered with a twist of humor, irony or provocation by contemporary spiritual teacher Lee Lozowick. They are compiled from twenty-five years of Lozowick's talks and seminars in the U.S., Canada, Europe, Mexico and India.

Paper, 150 pages, $12. 95   ISBN: 1-890772-21-6

YOUR BODY CAN TALK: *How to Use Simple Muscle Testing to Listen to What Your Body Knows and Needs*
by Susan L. Levy, D.C. and Carol Lehr, M.A.

Clear instructions in *simple muscle testing*, together with over 25 simple tests for how to use it for specific problems or disease conditions. Special chapters deal with health problems specific to women (especially PMS and Menopause) and problems specific to men (like stress, heart disease, and prostate difficulties). Contains over 30 diagrams, plus a complete Index and Resource Guide.

Paper, 350 pages, $19.95   ISBN: 0-934252-68-8

NATURAL HEALING WITH HERBS
by Humbart "Smokey" Santillo, N.D.
Foreword by Robert S. Mendelsohn, M.D.

Dr. Santillo's first book, and Hohm Press' long-standing best-seller, is a classic handbook on herbal and naturopathic treatment. Acclaimed as the most comprehensive work of its kind, *Natural Healing With Herbs* details (in layperson's terms) the properties and uses of 120 of the most common herbs and lists comprehensive therapies for more than 140 common ailments. All in alphabetical order for quick reference.
Over 150,000 copies in print.

Paper, 408 pages, $16.95   ISBN: 0-934252-08-4

To order: 1-800-381-2700 or visit our website www.hohmpress.com

FOOD ENZYMES: *The Missing Link To Radiant Health*
by Humbart "Smokey" Santillo, N.D.

Santillo's breakthrough book presents the most current research in this field, and encourages simple, straightforward steps for how to make enzyme supplementation a natural addition to a nutrition-conscious lifestyle. Special sections on: *Longevity and disease * The value of raw food and juicing * Detoxification * Prevention of allergies and candida * Sports and nutrition Over 200,000 copies in print.

Paper, 108 pages, U.S. $7.95   ISBN: 0-934252-40-8 (English)
Paper, 108 pages, U.S. $6.95   ISBN: 0-934252-49-1 (Spanish)
Audio version of *Food Enzymes*
2 cassette tapes, 150 minutes, U.S. $17.95,   ISBN: 0-934252-29-7

THE ROLFING EXPERIENCE: *Integration in the Gravity Field*
by Betsy Sise

Betsy Sise, a master Rolfer, certified in 1978, presents Ida Rolf's exciting work from the perspective of a long-time practitioner who has seen the miracles of both health and personal growth that it has effected in herself, her clients and those of others. Her book introduces the subject of Rolfing to the beginner in a form that is highly personal, and highly readable. She explains her own journey in training to be a Rolfer, presents an enticing overview of the basic philosophy of Ida Rolf's work, and leads the reader through a 10-session Rolfing series, answering the question, "What's it like to be Rolfed?"

Paper, 320 pages, $21.95   ISBN: 1-890772-52-6

To order: 1-800-381-2700 or visit our website www.hohmpress.com

YOU HAVE THE RIGHT TO REMAIN SILENT
Bringing Meditation to Life
by Rick Lewis

With sparkling clarity and humor, Rick Lewis explains exactly what meditation can offer to those who are ready to establish an island of sanity in the midst of an active life. This book is a comprehensive look at everything a beginner would need to start a meditation practice, including how to befriend an overactive mind and how to bring the fruits of meditation into all aspects of daily life. Experienced meditators will also find refreshing perspectives to both nourish and refine their practice.

Paper, 201 pages, $14.95   ISBN: 1-890772-23-2

TO TOUCH IS TO LIVE
The Need for Genuine Affection in an Impersonal World
by Mariana Caplan   Foreword by Ashley Montagu

The vastly impersonal nature of contemporary culture, supported by massive child abuse and neglect, and reinforced by growing techno-fascination are robbing us of our humanity. The author takes issue with the trends of the day that are mostly overlooked as being "progressive" or harmless, showing how these trends are actually undermining genuine affection and love. This uncompromising and inspiring work offers positive solutions for countering the effects of the growing depersonalization of our times.

"To all of us with bodies, in an increasingly disembodied world, this book comes as a passionate reminder that: Touch is essential to health and happiness."—Joanna Macy, author of *World as Lover, World as Self*

Paper, 384 pages, $19.95   ISBN: 1-890772-24-0

About the Author

C. Pierce Salguero graduated from the University of Virginia in 1996 as an anthropologist with a focus on Asia, and traveled to this part of the world shortly afterward. He soon fell in love with Thailand's unique culture and rich history, and what started as a short trip turned into a lengthy stay. Salguero lived and studied in Thailand from 1997 to 2001, researching Thai medical traditions and exploring an interest in Buddhism through extended stays at Thai meditation centers and monasteries. During this time he received training as a practitioner of massage and herbal medicine in Chiang Mai, Thailand, and apprenticed with individual folk healers. After returning to the U.S. he continued his formal studies at the University of Virginia and received an M.A. in East Asian Studies. His master's thesis was the basis for this book.

Pierce is currently the director of Tao Mountain Association of Traditional Thai Massage and Herbal Medicine, an educational resource for teachers, students, practitioners, and academic students of Thai healing methods. Tao Mountain's mission is to research, preserve, and educate about traditional Thai medicine as a serious traditional medical discipline. He is the author of *A Thai Herbal: Traditional Recipes for Health and Harmony* (2003), *The Encyclopedia of Thai Massage* (2004), *The Spiritual Healing of Traditional Thailand* (2005), and *The Encyclopedia of Thai Massage Student Workbook* (2007).

Contact Information
    See: www.taomountain.org
           www.jivaka.net
           www.shivago.org